Dental Radiography
A Workbook and Laboratory Manual

5th Edition

Joen M. Iannucci, DDS, MS
Professor of Clinical Dentistry
The Ohio State University
College of Dentistry
Columbus, Ohio

Laura Jansen Howerton, RDH, MS
Instructor
Wake Technical Community College
Raleigh, North Carolina

ELSEVIER

ELSEVIER

3251 Riverport Lane
St. Louis, Missouri 63043

Notices

Knowledge and best practice in this field are constantly changing. As new research and experience broaden our understanding, changes in research methods, professional practices, or medical treatment may become necessary.

Practitioners and researchers must always rely on their own experience and knowledge in evaluating and using any information, methods, compounds, or experiments described herein. In using such information or methods they should be mindful of their own safety and the safety of others, including parties for whom they have a professional responsibility.

With respect to any drug or pharmaceutical products identified, readers are advised to check the most current information provided (i) on procedures featured or (ii) by the manufacturer of each product to be administered, to verify the recommended dose or formula, the method and duration of administration, and contraindications. It is the responsibility of practitioners, relying on their own experience and knowledge of their patients, to make diagnoses, to determine dosages and the best treatment for each individual patient, and to take all appropriate safety precautions.

To the fullest extent of the law, neither the Publisher nor the authors, contributors, or editors, assume any liability for any injury and/or damage to persons or property as a matter of products liability, negligence or otherwise, or from any use or operation of any methods, products, instructions, or ideas contained in the material herein.

Content Strategist: Kristin Wilhelm
Content Development Manager: Ellen Wurm-Cutter
Content Development Specialist: John Tomedi, Spring Hollow Press
Publishing Services Manager: Hemamalini Rajendrababu
Project Manager: Radhika Sivalingam
Cover Designer: Muthukumaran Thangaraj

Printed in the United States of America

Last digit is the print number: 9   8   7   6   5   4   3   2

Working together
to grow libraries in
developing countries

www.elsevier.com • www.bookaid.org

To my Dad,
Angelo J. Iannucci

Thank you for making me the writer that I am today ---
without the Iannucci "writing & editing gene" *(inherited from you),*
this book would not be possible.

Thank you for always being there for me ---
for being my biggest fan, for making me laugh,
and, for always being the voice of reason.

Thank you for teaching me life's lessons ---
for showing me how to be independent,
and, for giving me wings to fly.

Thank you Dad,
for everything.

JMI

To the radiology faculty and staff members,
Thank you for continuing to learn from our students.

To the radiology students,
Thank you for keeping patient care number one.

LJH

Preface

Dental radiography is a required course for all dental assisting (DA) and dental hygiene (DH) programs. Dental imaging involves a high level of technical skill that cannot be learned in a lecture setting. To provide students with opportunities to apply concepts and practice techniques learned in the classroom, DA and DH programs include a laboratory component as part of the basic dental radiography course.

Dental Radiography: A Workbook and Laboratory Manual is a unique product designed to complement the core textbook Dental Radiography: Principles and Techniques, now in its fifth edition. When used together, these two products provide a direct link between classroom theory and clinical practice.

This workbook and laboratory manual is designed with *both* students *and* educators in mind. For the student, this workbook portion serves as an easy-to-follow road map that connects concepts and application. For the educator, the laboratory manual portion serves as a ready-to-go training resource for the hands-on component of a basic dental radiography course.

Dental Radiography: A Workbook and Laboratory Manual is an exciting new companion to the textbook, *Dental Radiography Principles and Techniques*. As it guides educators and students through core content, it provides an easy to use solution for teaching dental imaging techniques in DA and DH educational programs.

Joen M. Iannucci
Laura Jansen Howerton

Introduction

Dental Radiography: A Workbook and Laboratory Manual is arranged in two distinct sections.

The first section, the *Workbook*, is organized into seven modules that follow the seven parts of the companion textbook. This section contains:

- Vocabulary drills, short answer questions, and identification exercises to provide students with extra practice using newly learned terms and concepts
- Active learning experiences allowing students to develop hands-on knowledge and skills
- Critical thinking questions to help students apply what has just been learned to the practice setting
- "To do" checklists following each module to keep students organized
- Review materials that reinforce difficult material

The second section is structured as a *Laboratory Manual*, presenting the material and instructions needed for students to perform each of the dental imaging techniques. Through activities and assessments, students are first provided with a "tour" of the clinical laboratory environment. Then, students complete imaging techniques, first using the teaching manikin, followed by receptor placement practice with peers, in order to establish competency through active learning. Depending on educator preference, these technique activities can be used in any order and may be tailored to the specific needs of the DA or DH program.

For DA and DH programs with limited x-ray training equipment available, this workbook can be used by one group of students in the classroom, while another group participates in hands-on training in the clinical laboratory setting. Using these two sections, we've sought to create one turn-key manual that allows instructors to efficiently use dental radiography lab time to help students bridge theory and practice for clinical success.

Joen M. Iannucci
Laura Jansen Howerton

Reviewers

Sharron Cook, CDA
Instructor
Columbus Technical College
Columbus, Georgia

Amy E. Coplen, RDH, EPDH, MS
Associate Professor
Pacific University
Hillsboro, Oregon

Leslie Koberna, RDH, BSDH, MPH/HSA, PhD
Instructor, Dental Hygiene Program
Texas Women's University
Denton, Texas

Amy S. Rafter, RDH, RF, MSEd
Dental Hygiene Faculty
Century College
White Bear Lake, Minnesota

Janine Sasse-Englert, RDH, MS
Program Director, Dental Hygiene Program
Sheridan College
Sheridan, Wyoming

Contents

INSTRUCTIONS

How to Prepare
*   Review the learning objectives for Module 1 prior to lab.
*   Review the critical thinking questions for Module 1 prior to lab.

What to Bring
*   *Workbook and Laboratory Manual*—Module 1 materials
*   pencil
*   textbook (print or e-version)

Written Exercises
*   Work together or individually to complete each exercise.
*   For each chapter, complete the worksheets in pencil (*without looking up answers*).
*   When each exercise is finished, use your text to check answers; correct any wrong answers.
*   Use your completed and corrected packet to study for assessments.

Active Learning Experiences
*   Examine the lead apron and thyroid collar on display.
*   Practice placement of lead apron and thyroid collar on a classmate.
*   Examine collimators, aluminum disks and position indicating devices on display.
*   In pairs, take turns answering each critical thinking question and provide feedback to each other.
*   Ask your instructor to observe you answering the critical thinking questions and provide you with feedback.

Clinical Laboratory Activities
*   See Section 2, *Laboratory Manual,* Part 1 - Introduction to the Radiology Clinic.

Assessments
*   See Section 2, *Laboratory Manual,* Part 1 - Introduction to the Radiology Clinic

1 Radiation Basics

LEARNING OBJECTIVES

The goal of Module 1 is to provide students with a reinforcement of the fundamental understanding of radiation basics. Upon successful completion of Chapters 1 to 5 lectures and laboratory, the student will be able to:

CHAPTER	LEARNING OBJECTIVES
CHAPTER 1 RADIATION HISTORY	
Written Exercises	• Define basic terminology used in dental imaging. • Identify who discovered x-rays and what year the discovery took place. • Discuss the importance of dental images. • List the uses of dental images.
CHAPTER 2 RADIATION PHYSICS	
Written Exercises	• Define basic terminology used in radiation physics. • Identify and label the parts of the dental x-ray machine and x-ray tubehead. • Identify and label the parts of the x-ray tube; describe how dental x-rays are produced within the x-ray tube. • Identify the properties of x-radiation. • Identify and label each component part of the dental x-ray tubehead.
CHAPTER 3 RADIATION CHARACTERISTICS	
Written Exercises	• Define basic terminology used with radiation characteristics. • Recognize and discuss scales of contrast. • Recognize how kV, mA, and exposure time affect the x-ray beam and resultant image. • State the useful range of kV and mA used in dental imaging. • State the formula for the inverse square law and explain radiation intensity.
CHAPTER 4 RADIATION BIOLOGY	
Written Exercises	• Define basic terminology used with radiation biology. • Define radiation injury factors and radiation effects. • List the units of measurement used in radiation exposure. • Identify tissues/organs as radioresistant or radiosensitive. • Define the risks vs. benefits of dental images and list ways to limit patient exposure.

CHAPTER 5   RADIATION PROTECTION

Written Exercises	• Define basic terminology used with radiation protection. • List and describe ways to protect a patient before, during, and after radiation exposure. • Discuss operator protection in terms of distance, shielding, and positioning. • Define MPD, cumulative occupational dose, and ALARA.

MODULE 1   ACTIVE LEARNING EXPERIENCES

	• Identify lead apron and shielding as ways to limit x-ray exposure. • Practice lead apron placement on classmates. • Practice explaining the use of the lead apron as you place the lead apron on a classmate. • Practice answering questions concerning the lead apron. • Identify collimators, aluminum disks, and position indicating devices (PIDs).

MODULE 1   CLINICAL LABORATORY ACTIVITIES

	• Apply information learned to complete activities in Section 2, *Laboratory Manual*, Part 1 - Introduction to the Radiology Clinic *(as assigned by instructor).*

MODULE 1   ASSESSMENTS

	• Apply information learned to complete assessments in Section 2, *Laboratory Manual*, Part 1 - Introduction to the Radiology Clinic *(as assigned by instructor).*

WORKBOOK EXERCISES

Chapter 1   Radiation History

BASIC TERMINOLOGY CROSSWORD PUZZLE

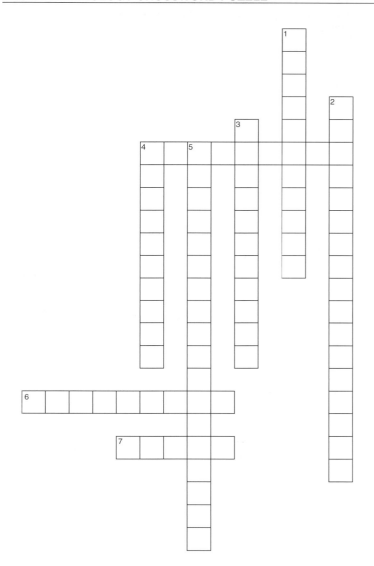

DOWN

1   a high-energy radiation produced by the collision of a beam of electrons with a metal target in an x-ray tube

2   the production of radiographs of the teeth and adjacent structures by the exposure of film to x-rays

3   the art and science of making radiographs by the exposure of film to x-rays

4   a picture (visible photographic record) on film produced by the passage of x-rays through an object or body

5   any person who positions and exposes dental receptors

ACROSS

4   a form of energy carried by waves or a stream of particles

6   the science or study of radiation as used in medicine

7   a beam of energy that has the power to penetrate substances and record image shadows on receptors

COMPLETION AND SHORT ANSWER

History Highlights

1. _____ discovered x-rays.

2. X-rays were discovered in the year _____.

3. Describe the history of x-ray film.

   _____

   _____

   _____

   _____

Importance of Dental Images

1. _____ is one of the most important uses of dental images.

2. Briefly state the importance of dental images.

   _____

   _____

   _____

   _____

Uses of Dental Images

Refer to Box 1.1 of your textbook to answer the questions below.

1. Dental images are used to detect lesions, diseases, and conditions of teeth and surrounding structures that _____

   _____.

2. Dental images are used to confirm or classify _____.

3. Dental images are used to _____ lesions or foreign objects.

4. Dental images are used to provide information during _____.

5. Dental images are used to evaluate _____ and _____.

6. Dental images are used to illustrate changes secondary to _____, _____ _____, and _____.

7. Dental images are used to document the condition of a patient _____.

8. Dental images are used to aid in the development of a _____.

ORDERING

Highlights in Dental Imaging History

Arrange the following in order of discovery from earliest to latest.

_____ 1. Introduction of panoramic imaging

_____ 2. Introduction of the bite-wing technique

_____ 3. Introduction of intraoral digital imaging

_____ 4. Introduction of cone-beam computed tomography (CBCT)

_____ 5. First dental x-ray machine

_____ 6. Introduction of F-speed film

_____ 7. First dental radiograph

WORKBOOK EXERCISES

Chapter 2   Radiation Physics

BASIC TERMINOLOGY CROSSWORD PUZZLE

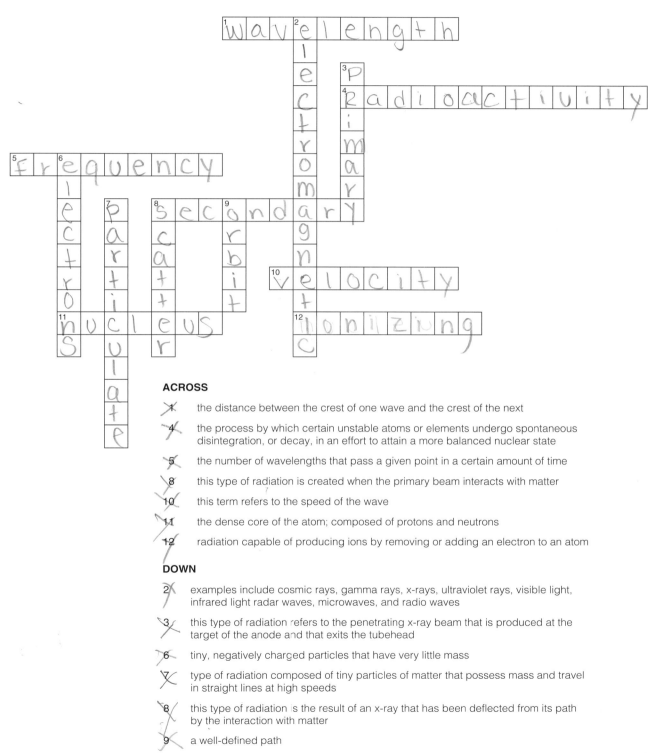

ACROSS

1   the distance between the crest of one wave and the crest of the next

4   the process by which certain unstable atoms or elements undergo spontaneous disintegration, or decay, in an effort to attain a more balanced nuclear state

5   the number of wavelengths that pass a given point in a certain amount of time

8   this type of radiation is created when the primary beam interacts with matter

10   this term refers to the speed of the wave

11   the dense core of the atom; composed of protons and neutrons

12   radiation capable of producing ions by removing or adding an electron to an atom

DOWN

2   examples include cosmic rays, gamma rays, x-rays, ultraviolet rays, visible light, infrared light radar waves, microwaves, and radio waves

3   this type of radiation refers to the penetrating x-ray beam that is produced at the target of the anode and that exits the tubehead

6   tiny, negatively charged particles that have very little mass

7   type of radiation composed of tiny particles of matter that possess mass and travel in straight lines at high speeds

8   this type of radiation is the result of an x-ray that has been deflected from its path by the interaction with matter

9   a well-defined path

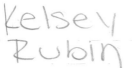
Kelsey Rubin

IDENTIFICATION AND LABELING

Dental X-Ray Machine

Identify each item in Fig. 2-1.

1. Identify A _Control panel_

2. Identify B _extension arm_

3. Identify C _tubehead_

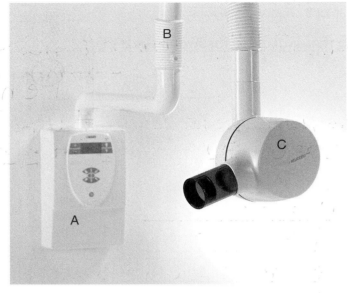

Fig. 2-1 (Courtesy Sirona Dental USA Inc., Charlotte, NC.)

Dental X-Ray Tubehead

Identify each item in Fig. 2-2.

1. _X-ray tubehead_

2. _Position-indicating device_

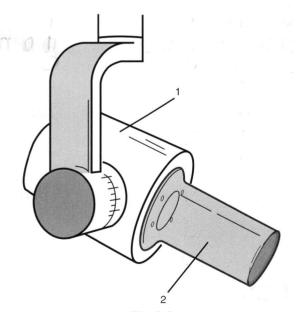

Fig. 2-2

10

Dental X-Ray Tube

Identify each item in Fig. 2-3.

1. Focal spot on tungsten target
2. Glass envelope
3. Vacuum
4. Copper stem
5. Anode (+)
6. Useful x-ray beam
7. tube window
8. Cathode (-)
9. electronic focusing cup
10. Filament + electron cloud

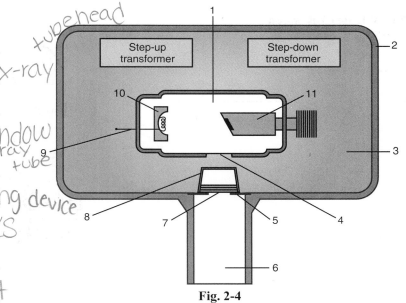

Fig. 2-3

Dental X-Ray Tubehead

Identify each item in Fig. 2-4.

1. X-ray tube
2. metal housing of x-ray
3. Insulating oil
4. Unleaded glass window of x-ray tube
5. lead collimator
6. Position-indicating device
7. Aluminum disks
8. tubehead seal
9. Filament circuit
10. Cathode (-)
11. Anode (+)

Step-up transformer   Step-down transformer

tubehead

Fig. 2-4

Kelsey Rubin

SHORT ANSWER

Production of Dental X-Rays

1. Describe the production of x-rays in the x-ray tube illustrated in Fig. 2-5.

A. When filament circuit is activated, the filament heats up, and thermionic emission occurs.

B. When the exposure button is activated, the electrons are accelerated from the cathode to the anode

C. The electrons strike the tungsten target, and their kinetic energy is converted to x-rays and heat.

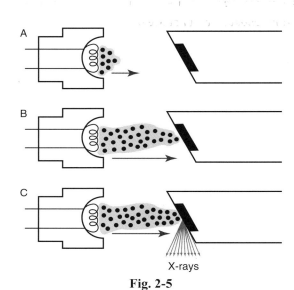

X-rays

Fig. 2-5

2. Describe how **"cat → nap"** can help you to remember the flow of the electrons in the x-ray tube.

CAT = cathode   electrons travel from
NAP = negative   cathode -> anodes
A = anode
P = positive

MULTIPLE CHOICE

Properties of X-Rays

Circle each correct answer.

1. **appearance**   X-rays are **visible** / **(invisible.)**
2. **mass**   X-rays have **weight** / **(no weight.)**
3. **charge**   X-rays have **(no charge)** / **+ charge** / **– charge.**
4. **speed**   X-rays travel at the **(speed of sound)** / **speed of light.**
5. **wavelength**   X-rays have **long** / **(short)** wavelengths with a **(high)** / **low** frequency.
6. **path of travel**   X-rays travel in straight lines and **can** / **(cannot)** be deflected.
7. **focusing capability**   X-rays **can** / **(cannot)** be focused to a point.
8. **penetrating power**   X-rays **(can)** / **cannot** penetrate liquids, solids, and gases.
9. **absorption**   X-rays **(are)** / **are not** absorbed by matter.
10. **ionization**   X-rays **(cause)** / **do not cause** ionization.
11. **fluorescence**   X-rays **(can)** / **cannot** cause certain substances to fluoresce.
12. **effect on film**   X-rays **(can)** / **cannot** produce an image on photographic film.
13. **effect on tissues**   X-rays **(cause)** / **do not cause** biologic changes in living cells.

WORKBOOK EXERCISES

Chapter 3 Radiation Characteristics

BASIC TERMINOLOGY CROSSWORD PUZZLE

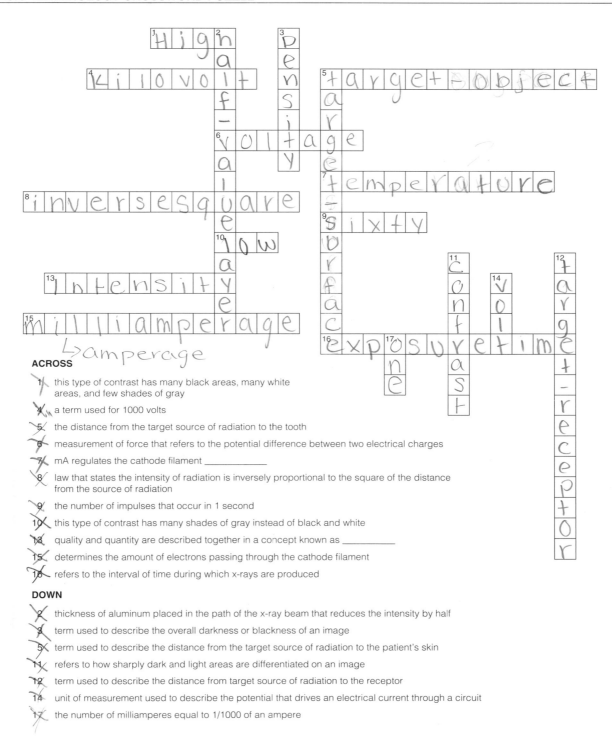

Crossword answers filled in:
1. High
2. half-value
3. density
4. kilovolt
5. target-object / target
6. voltage
7. temperature
8. inversesquare
9. sixty
10. low
11. contrast
12. target-receptor
13. intensity
14. volt
15. milliamperage (amperage)
16. exposuretime
17. one

ACROSS

1. this type of contrast has many black areas, many white areas, and few shades of gray
4. a term used for 1000 volts
5. the distance from the target source of radiation to the tooth
6. measurement of force that refers to the potential difference between two electrical charges
7. mA regulates the cathode filament _____
8. law that states the intensity of radiation is inversely proportional to the square of the distance from the source of radiation
9. the number of impulses that occur in 1 second
10. this type of contrast has many shades of gray instead of black and white
13. quality and quantity are described together in a concept known as _____
15. determines the amount of electrons passing through the cathode filament
16. refers to the interval of time during which x-rays are produced

DOWN

2. thickness of aluminum placed in the path of the x-ray beam that reduces the intensity by half
3. term used to describe the overall darkness or blackness of an image
5. term used to describe the distance from the target source of radiation to the patient's skin
11. refers to how sharply dark and light areas are differentiated on an image
12. term used to describe the distance from target source of radiation to the receptor
14. unit of measurement used to describe the potential that drives an electrical current through a circuit
17. the number of milliamperes equal to 1/1000 of an ampere

Kelsey Rubin

MULTIPLE CHOICE

Contrast

Circle the correct answer.

1. low contrast = **long / short** scale contrast = **many / few** shades of gray

2. high contrast = **long / short** scale contrast = **many / few** shades of gray

3. short-scale contrast results from **low / high** kV

4. long-scale contrast results from **low / high** kV

SELECT ALL THAT APPLY

Exposure Factors and Density

Place a check mark (✔) for each that applies.

1. An image that is **dark** (increased density) may result from:

   ✓ kV too high

   ✓ mA too high

   ✓ too much exposure time

   _____ too little exposure time

   _____ kV too low

   _____ mA too low

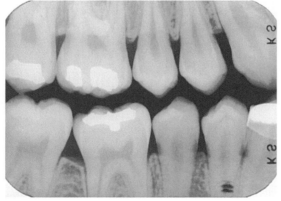

Diagnostic image

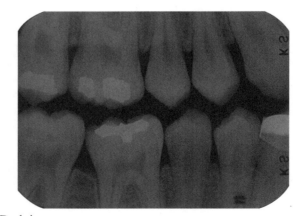

Dark image

2. An image that is **light** (decreased density) may result from:

_____ kV too high

_____ mA too high

_____ too much exposure time

√ too little exposure time

√ kV too low

√ mA too low

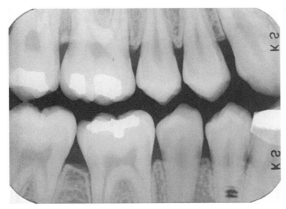

Diagnostic image

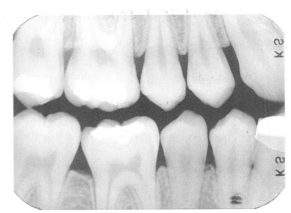

Light image

COMPLETION

Contrast

Identify whether the image is high contrast or low contrast.

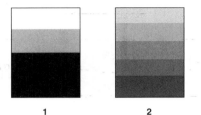

1
2

1. *high contrast*
2. *low contrast*

Range of kV and mA

1. The range of kV currently used in dental imaging is *65* to *100*.

2. The range of mA currently used in dental imaging is *6* to *8*.

Distances

Name each of the distances indicated in the diagram below.

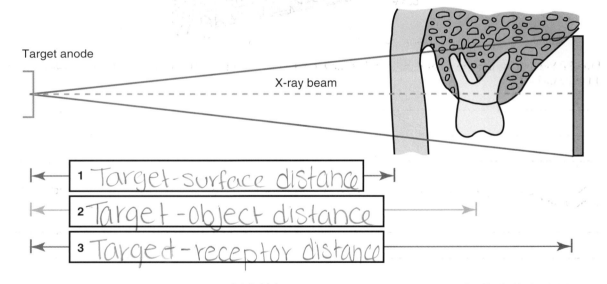

Target anode

X-ray beam

1 *Target-surface distance*

2 *Target-object distance*

3 *Target-receptor distance*

Kelsey Rubin

SHORT ANSWER

X-Ray Beam Quality and Quantity

1. Describe how kilovoltage and milliamperage relate to x-ray beam quality and quantity.

the quality is controled by Kilovoltage while quantity is controled by milliamperage

2. Describe how using the beam from a flashlight can help you remember the relationship between distance and intensity.

x-rays travel away from their source of origin, the intensity of the beam lessens

Inverse Square Law

The Inverse Square Rule

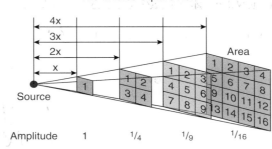

1. If the PID length is changed from 8 to 16 inches, how does the increase in target-receptor distance affect the intensity of the beam?

doubleing the distance frome the source of radiation to the receptor results in a beam that is one fourth as intense.

2. If the PID length is changed from 16 to 8 inches, how does the decrease in target-receptor distance affect the intensity of the beam?

it decreases the distance in half making the beam 2x more intense.

3. State the formula used to calculate the inverse square law.

$$\frac{\text{original intensity}}{\text{New intensity}} = \frac{\text{New distance}^2}{\text{Original distance}^2}$$

19

WORKBOOK EXERCISES

Chapter 4   Radiation Biology

BASIC TERMINOLOGY CROSSWORD PUZZLE

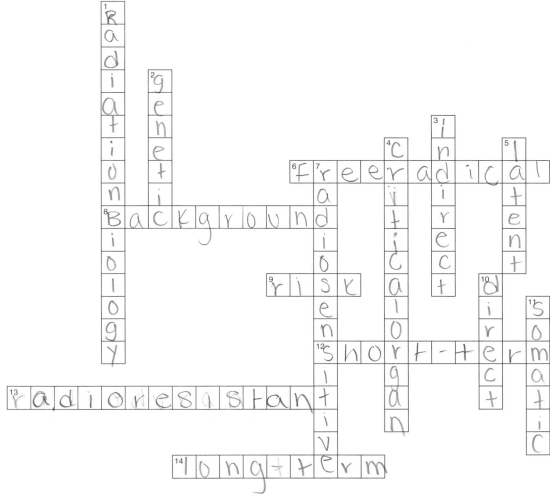

Crossword solution:
- 1 Down: Radiationbiology
- 2 Down: genetic
- 3 Down: indirect
- 4 Down: critical organ
- 5 Down: latent
- 6 Across: Free radical
- 8 Across: Background
- 9 Across: risk
- 10 Down: direct
- 11 Down: somatic
- 12 Across: short-term
- 13 Across: radioresistant
- 14 Across: long term

ACROSS

6 uncharged atom or molecule with a single, unpaired electron in its outermost shell

8 a type of ionizing radiation that is ubiquitous in the environment

9 the likelihood of adverse effects or death resulting from exposure to a hazard

12 radiation effects that follow the latent period and are seen within minutes, days, or weeks

13 cell that is resistant to radiation

14 radiation effects that follow the latent period and are seen years or generations later

DOWN

1 study of the effects of ionizing radiation on living tissue

2 type of cell that includes reproductive cells

3 a theory of radiation injury that suggests x-rays are absorbed and form toxins which damage the cell

4 if damaged, dimishes the quality of a person's life

5 a period of time that elapses between exposure to ionizing radiation and appearance of observable clinical signs

7 cell that is sensitive to radiation

10 a theory of injury that suggests damage results when ionizing radiation directly hits critical areas within the cell

11 type of cells that include all cells in the body except reproductive

Kelsey Rubin

COMPLETION AND SHORT ANSWER

Radiation Injury Factors

1. **Total dose:** more damage occurs when tissues absorb __large__ quantities of radiation.

2. **Dose rate:** more damage takes place with __high__ dose rates because repair cannot take place.

3. **Amount irradiated:** more damage occurs when __large__ amounts of the body are exposed to radiation.

4. **Cell sensitivity:** more damage occurs in cells that are more __sensitive__ to radiation.

5. **Age:** persons who are __children__ are more susceptible to damage than persons who are __adults__.

6. **Stochastic effects:** the severity of the response is __direct function__ of the dose.

7. **Non-stochastic effects:** the severity of the effect increases with __larger__ dose.

8. List examples of **stochastic effects**. __leukemia and other cancers i.e. tumors__

9. List examples of **non-stochastic effects**. __skin erythema, loss of hair, cataract formation, decreased fertility, radiation sickness etc.__

10. List the events in the **sequence of radiation injury**. __latent period, period of injury, and recovery period__

Radiation Effects

1. **Short-term effects** are associated with __large__ amounts of radiation absorbed in a __short__ period of time.

2. List examples of **short-term effects**. __acute radiation syndrome, vomitting, diarrhea, hair loss__

3. **Long-term effects** are associated with __small__ amounts of radiation absorbed in a __long__ period of time.

4. List examples of **long-term effects**. __cancer, birth abnormalities, and genetic effects__

Identify the labeled mutations in Fig. 4-1 as genetic or somatic.

5. Identify A _Genetic mutation_

6. Identify B _Somatic mutation_

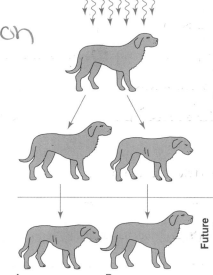

Risk vs. Benefit

1. When dental images are properly prescribed and exposed, the benefit of ___disease detection___ outweighs the risk of ___biologic damage___

IDENTIFICATION

Radiation Effects on Tissues and Organs

Identify each tissue/organ listed as either RR (radioresistant) or RS (radiosensitive). Place an **X** near the three most sensitive tissues/organs. Place a check mark (✔) near the two most resistant tissues/organs.

1. __X__ bone marrow

2. _____ intestinal mucosa

3. _____ salivary gland

4. _____ lens of eye

5. _____ kidney

6. _____ oral mucosa

7. _____ liver

8. __X__ reproductive cells

9. __✓__ mature bone and cartilage

10. __✓__ nerve tissue

11. _____ skin

12. _____ thyroid gland

13. __X__ small lymphocyte

14. __✓__ muscle tissue

Kelsey
Rubin

COMPLETION AND SHORT ANSWER

Radiation Measurements

Name the radiation units of measurement in both the traditional and SI systems.

Traditional system

1. <u>Roentgen (R)</u> exposure
2. <u>Radiation absorbed dose (rad)</u> dose
3. <u>Roentgen equivalent in man (rem)</u> dose equivalent

SI system

1. <u>Gray (Gy)</u> dose
2. <u>Sievert (Sv)</u> dose equivalent

Patient Exposure and Dose

List four of the six ways to limit patient exposure to x-radiation.

1. <u>Collimation</u>
2. <u>lead apron</u>
3. <u>thyroid collar</u>
4. <u>Position-indicating device (PID)</u>

Name *Kelsey Rubin*

Date _____

WORKBOOK EXERCISES

Chapter 5   Radiation Protection

BASIC TERMINOLOGY CROSSWORD PUZZLE

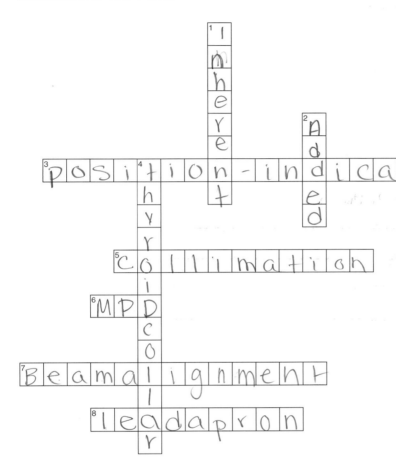

ACROSS

3. extension of the x-ray tubehead; is used to direct the x-ray beam

5. used to restrict size and shape of x-ray beam and to reduce patient exposure

6. maximum dose equivalent that a body is permitted to receive in a specific period of time

7. a device that helps to stabilize the receptor position in the mouth and reduces the chances of movement

8. a flexible shield placed over the patient's chest and lap to protect the reproductive and blood-forming tissues from scatter radiation

DOWN

1. type of filtration in the x-ray tubehead that includes the glass window of the x-ray tube, the insulating oil, and tubehead seal

2. type of filtration that consists of alumimum disks placed in the path of the x-ray beam between collimator and tubehead seal

4. flexible lead shield that is placed securely around patient's neck to protect thyroid gland from scatter

Kelsey Rubin

IDENTIFICATION, LABELING, AND SHORT ANSWER

Patient and Operator Protection

1. Identify the part of the tubehead labeled in Fig. 5-1.

   Aluminum Filtration disk

2. State the purpose of this part of the tubehead.

   To filter out the nonpenertrating, longer wavelength x-rays. thickness from .5mm to 2.0mm.

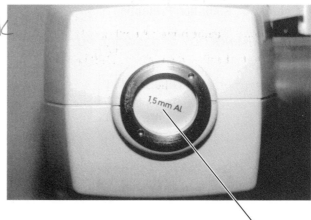

Fig. 5-1

3. Identify the part of the tubehead labeled in Fig. 5-2.

   lead collimator

4. State the purpose of this part of the tubehead.

   fits over the opening, circle or rectangle, and restricts the size of the x-ray beam

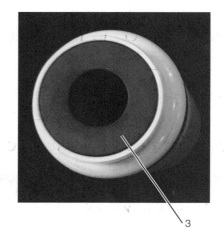

Fig. 5-2

5. Federal regulations require that the diameter of a collimated x-ray beam be restricted to ___2.75___ inches at the patient's skin.

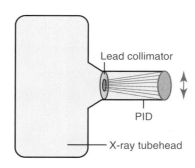

Lead collimator

PID

X-ray tubehead

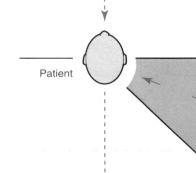

X-ray tubehead

Primary beam

Patient

Radiographer

6. The dental radiographer should stand at least __6__ feet from the x-ray tubehead.

7. The dental radiographer should stand perpendicular to the beam or at a __90__-degree to __135__-degree angle to the beam.

Radiation Exposure Guidelines

1. Define **MPD**. The maximum permissible dose rise defined by the NCRR as the maximum dose equivalent that a body is premitted to recieve in within a specific period

2. State the MPD for **occupationally exposed persons**: __50__ mSv/year

3. State the MPD for **nonoccupationally exposed persons**: __1__ mSv/year

4. Define **cumulative occupational dose**. The occupationally exposed workers must not exceed an accumutated lifetime radiation does

5. List the **cumulative occupational dose** for a person who is 35 years old. 350 mSv (0.5 Sv)

6. Define **ALARA**. "as low as resonably achievable" concept states that all exposure to radiation must be kept to a minmum.

7. Discuss the importance of using a **lead apron and thyroid collar** to protect a patient from excess radiation exposure. The lead apron prevents the radiation from reaching these radiosensitive organs. And the collar prevents scatter radiation from reaching the highly radiosensitive tissues of the thyroid.

27

Kelsey Rubin

APPLICATION

Module 1 Radiation Basics

SELF-ASSESSMENT

Chapters 1 - 5

Based on the worksheets that you have just completed for Chapters 1 - 5, how prepared are you for assessments?

_____ very prepared, confident

_____ somewhat prepared, somewhat confident

___X___ somewhat unprepared, lack confidence

_____ unprepared, no confidence

Based on your answer above, what is your plan for improvement? List the topics and concepts that you need to further review and study for assessments.

I was looking back at the chapters a lot
for answers, so I need to write out
the words + define them as well as maybe
read them again.

CRITICAL THINKING QUESTIONS

What does all the information in Chapters 1 to 5 mean to you in the practice setting? Use the questions below to help you apply the information that you have just learned. Work in pairs and practice answering these questions with your classmates. Share feedback concerning the content and delivery of information—is the information correct and understandable for the average patient? Are effective communication skills being used? The more you practice, the more comfortable you will be discussing these issues with your patients.

1. **You explain to a new patient that it is necessary to take dental images at her new patient appointment. The patient shows signs of concern and asks why it is necessary to have x-rays taken.**

   How will you respond to this patient?

   • CHAPTER 1—see importance of dental x-rays and uses of dental images

2. **A 40-year-old man comes to your office for a new patient examination. The patient reports not having been to the dentist for the past 8 years. He claims to brush his teeth one time per day but does not floss. He complains that a few of his teeth have recently become sensitive to hot and cold. After the oral examination, the dentist orders a complete series of images. While you are preparing the necessary receptors and holders, the patient asks "why do you need to take so many x-rays?"**

   How will you respond to this patient?

   • CHAPTER 1—see uses of dental images

   • CHAPTER 5—see guidelines for prescribing dental images; see radiation protection and patient education

3. **Your office has just reopened after being closed for the holidays. You have been asked to retake an image that you just took on a patient because the dentist states that, although you captured the correct tooth, it is of non-diagnostic quality: the film is far too light.**

   What exposure factors will you check in order to assure the second exposure is of diagnostic quality?

   • CHAPTER 3—see how adjustment of kV, mA, and time can affect the density of an image

4. **A 43-year-old woman calls your office and wants to become a new patient. She states that she has not been to the dentist in over 5 years, and she is experiencing pain and discomfort. She wants to schedule an appointment to see the dentist. You explain to her that her first visit will consist of a comprehensive examination and a series of x-rays, but she appears apprehensive and is asking a lot of questions. She wants to know why you need to take x-rays, if dental x-rays are safe, and how many will be taken.**

   How will you respond to this patient?

   • CHAPTER 1—see uses of dental images

   • CHAPTER 4—see how ionizing radiation is harmful; see risks vs. benefits

   • CHAPTER 5—see guidelines for prescribing dental images; see radiation protection and patient education

5. **A new patient in your office is told that she is in need of a complete series of x-rays. She is concerned about the risks with taking so many x-rays. The patient asks you for more background information regarding radiation exposure. How will you respond to this patient?**

   • CHAPTER 4—see radiation exposure, risks vs. benefits, and patient dose information

6. **You are assisting the dentist with a new patient, a 35-year-old woman. She has a large swelling associated with a lower left molar and has not been able to sleep or eat for the past 2 days because of the pain associated with her tooth. The dentist orders an image of the area. Once the dentist leaves the room, the patient becomes reluctant to have the image taken because of the exposure to radiation. How will you respond to this patient? What information can you share with this patient concerning the protection steps that will be used before, during, and after x-ray exposure?**

- CHAPTER 1—see importance of dental x-rays and uses of dental images

- CHAPTER 4—see radiation exposure, risks vs. benefits, and patient dose information

- CHAPTER 5—see radiation protection before, during, and after exposure; see radiation protection and patient education

7. **As you are placing a lead apron and thyroid collar on your patient prior to beginning exposures of dental images, the patient asks the following questions:**

    - My last dentist never used a lead apron, was that wrong?

    - My child's dentist does not use an apron. Should I request one?

    - Why is this so high around my neck?

   How will you respond to this patient?

8. **Your dentist employer wants everyone in the office to deliver a uniform message to patients about lead apron use and how exposure to dental x-rays is limited. She asks you to prepare an example dialogue and present it to the office staff for their use with patients.**

   What will you prepare to present to the office staff?

TO-DO CHECKLIST

Written Exercises

_____ Complete all worksheets.

_____ Complete self-assessment.

Active Learning Experiences

_____ Examine the collimators, aluminum disks and position indicating devices on display.

_____ Examine the lead apron and thyroid collar on display.

_____ Practice the placement of lead apron and thyroid collar on a classmate.

_____ Review and answer the critical thinking questions.

_____ Practice answering critical thinking questions with your classmates and provide feedback.

Clinical Laboratory Activities

_____ Complete activities in Section 2, _Laboratory Manual_, Part 1 - Introduction to the Radiology Clinic _(as assigned by instructor)_.

Assessments

_____ Complete assessments in Section 2, _Laboratory Manual_, Part 1 - Introduction to the Radiology Clinic _(as assigned by instructor)_.

NUMBERS REVIEW

CHAPTER 1

1895	**x-rays discovered** by Wilhelm Roentgen
1923	**first dental x-ray unit**
2%	exposure time today is **<2% of exposure time used in 1920**

CHAPTER 2

99%	in x-ray tube, amount of energy **lost as heat**
01%	in x-ray tube, amount of energy **converted to x-rays**
3 to 5 volts	used in low-voltage filament circuit; controlled by **mA**
65,000 to 100,000 V	volts used in high-voltage circuit, controlled by **kV**
70%	of x-ray energy produced is **general radiation** (braking)
62%	of x-ray beam interaction with matter is **Compton scatter**
30%	of x-ray beam interaction with matter is **photoelectric effect**
0.08%	of x-ray beam interaction with matter is **coherent scatter**

CHAPTER 3

Kilovolt	= **1000** volts
Milliampere	= **1/1000** of an ampere
Impulse	= **1/60** of a second
60 impulses	= **1** second
60 to 70 kV	**range of kV** currently used in dental imaging
6 to 8 mA	**range of mA** currently used in dental imaging
¼ as intense	results when PID length is **doubled (from 8 to 16 inches)**
4 times as intense	results when PID length is **halved (from 16 to 8 inches)**

CHAPTER 4

1 Gy	= 100 rad
1 rad	= 0.01 Gy
1 Sv	= 100 rem
1 rem	= 0.01 Sv
1 R = 1 rad = 1 rem	
1 Gy = 1 Sv	
3 in 1 million	risk of **dental imaging inducing a fatal cancer**
3300 in 1 million	risk of **spontaneously developing a fatal cancer**
60%	when using **rectangular** instead of round collimation, **60% less tissue is exposed**
60%	reduction of exposure when using **F-speed instead of D-speed film**

2.5 mm	amount of **total** aluminum filtration required **≥ 70kVp**
2.75 inches	size of **diameter of collimated beam** at patient's skin; collimated beam cannot exceed 2.75 inches
6 feet	**minimum required distance** of operator from primary beam
90 to 135 degrees	radiographer must stand **at an angle of 90 to 135 degrees to the primary beam**
0.25 mm	**minimum thickness of lead** or lead equivalent to provide protection (as in a lead apron)
50 mSv/year	**MPD** for **occupationally** exposed person = 0.050 Sv/year
0.5 mSv/month	**MPD for pregnant dental personnel** during pregnancy months
1 mSv/year	**MPD** for **nonoccupationally** exposed person
10 mSv/year	**cumulative occupational dose**; this is the lifetime limit of an occupationally exposed person; worker's age x **10 mSv/year** = cumulative occupational dose

WAVELENGTH REVIEW

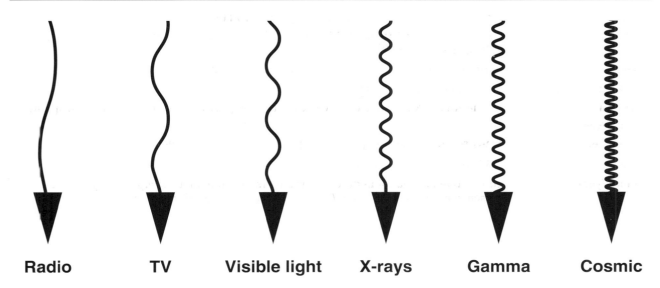

Radio **TV** **Visible light** **X-rays** **Gamma** **Cosmic**

- Which has the shortest wavelength?
- Which has the longest wavelength?

- Which has the lowest frequency?
- Which has the highest frequency?

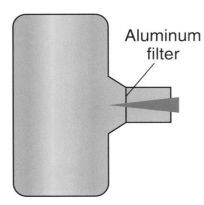

Aluminum filter

- Which is **most** penetrating?
- Which is **least** penetrating?

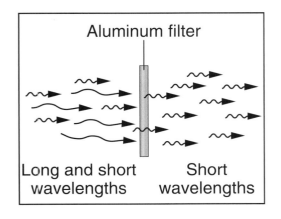

Aluminum filter

Long and short wavelengths

Short wavelengths

long wavelength / **lazy**
short wavelength / **strong**

HOW TO REMEMBER the difference between...
- high contrast & low contrast
- short-scale contrast & long-scale contrast

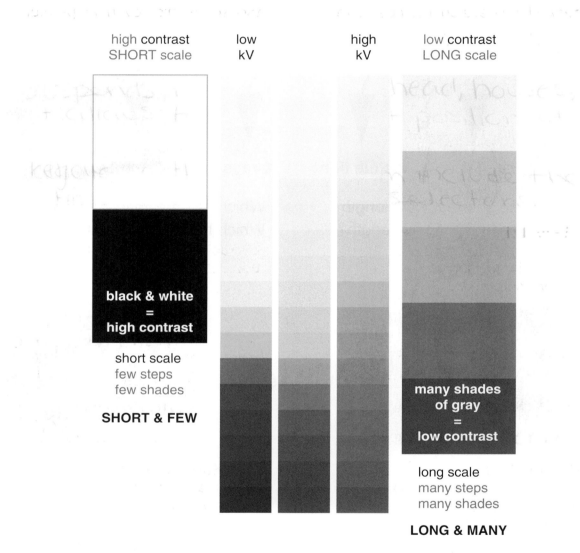

high contrast
SHORT scale

low
kV

high
kV

low contrast
LONG scale

black & white
=
high contrast

short scale
few steps
few shades

SHORT & FEW

many shades
of gray
=
low contrast

long scale
many steps
many shades

LONG & MANY

IMAGE DENSITY REVIEW

Dental images are sometimes too light or too dark. To remember the causes, think of how time and temperature affects the baking of cookies.

IMAGE - too dark
too much / high developer temperature
too much time in developer
too much kV and/or mA

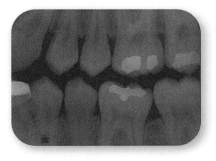

IMAGE - just right
correct developer temperature
correct time in developer
correct kV and/or mA

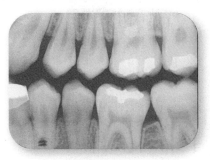

IMAGE - too light
too little / low developer temperature
too little time in developer
too little kV and/or mA

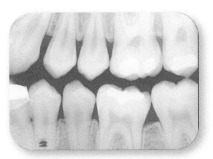

COOKIES - too dark
too much / high oven temperature
too much time in oven

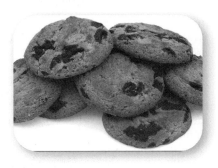

COOKIES - just right
correct oven temperature
correct time in oven

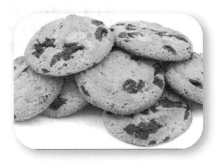

COOKIES - too light
too little / low oven temperature
too little time in oven

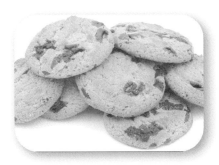

MODULE 2   EQUIPMENT, FILM, AND PROCESSING BASICS

INSTRUCTIONS

How to Prepare
- Review the learning objectives for Module 2 prior to lab.
- Review the critical thinking questions for Module 2 prior to lab.

What to Bring
- *Workbook and Laboratory Manual*—Module 2 materials
- pencil
- textbook (print or e-version)

Written Exercises
- Work together or individually to complete each exercise.
- For each chapter, complete the worksheets in pencil (*without looking up answers*).
- When each exercise is finished, use your text to check answers; correct any wrong answers.
- Use your completed and corrected packet to study for assessments.

Active Learning Experiences
- Identify and assemble RINN devices.
- Complete the shadow casting exercises.
- Identify the parts of the intraoral film packet, sizes of film, bite-wing tab, extraoral film, intensifying screen, and cassette.
- In pairs, take turns answering each critical thinking question and provide feedback to each other.
- Ask your instructor to observe you answering the critical thinking questions and provide you with feedback.

Clinical Laboratory Activities
- See Section 2, *Laboratory Manual,* Part 1 - Introduction to the Radiology Clinic.

Assessments
- See Section 2, *Laboratory Manual,* Part 1 - Introduction to the Radiology Clinic.

2 Equipment, Film, and Processing Basics

LEARNING OBJECTIVES

The goal of Module 2 laboratory experiences is to provide students with a reinforcement of the fundamental understanding of equipment, film and processing basics. Upon successful completion of Chapters 6 to 10 lectures and laboratory, the student will be able to:

CHAPTER	LEARNING OBJECTIVES
CHAPTER 6 DENTAL X-RAY EQUIPMENT	
Written Exercises	• Define basic terminology used with dental x-ray equipment. • Describe the dental x-ray machine component parts and explain the function of each. • Describe the purposes of a receptor holder/beam alignment device.
Active Learning Experiences	• Identify the parts of the RINN devices. • Assemble RINN devices.
CHAPTER 7 DENTAL X-RAY FILM	
Written Exercises	• Define basic terminology used with dental x-ray film. • Detail film composition and latent image formation. • List and describe the different types of intraoral and extraoral films available. • Describe duplicating film; identify and discuss intensifying screens and cassettes. • Discuss film storage and protection.
Active Learning Experiences	• Identify the following: parts of the intraoral film packet, sizes of intraoral film, bite-wing tab, extraoral film, intensifying screen, and cassette.
CHAPTER 8 DENTAL X-RAY IMAGE CHARACTERISTICS	
Written Exercises	• Define basic terminology used with image characteristics. • Define radiolucent and radiopaque, identify examples of each, and describe a diagnostic image. • Describe in detail the visual and geometric characteristics of radiographic images. • List the factors that affect sharpness, magnification, and distortion. • Review scales of contrast and how kV, mA, and exposure time affect an image (from Module 1).
Active Learning Experiences	• Complete shadow casting activities.
CHAPTER 9 DENTAL X-RAY FILM PROCESSING	
Written Exercises	• Define basic terminology used with film processing. • Briefly describe automatic processing; discuss advantages and disadvantages. • Discuss the lighting and equipment necessary for a darkroom. • Identify processing problems and discuss solutions.

CHAPTER 10   QUALITY ASSURANCE IN THE DENTAL OFFICE

Written Exercises

- Define basic terminology used with quality assurance.
- List examples of quality control tests for dental x-ray equipment, supplies, and processing.
- Identify how often quality control tests should be performed for dental x-ray machines, film, screens, cassettes, processing equipment, solutions, and view boxes.

MODULE 2   CLINICAL LABORATORY ACTIVITIES

- Apply information learned to complete activities in Section 2, *Laboratory Manual*, Part 1 - Introduction to the Radiology Clinic *(as assigned by instructor)*.

MODULE 2   ASSESSMENTS

- Apply information learned to complete assessments in Section 2, *Laboratory Manual*, Part 1 - Introduction to the Radiology Clinic *(as assigned by instructor)*.

WORKBOOK EXERCISES

Chapter 6 Dental X-Ray Equipment

BASIC TERMINOLOGY CROSSWORD PUZZLE

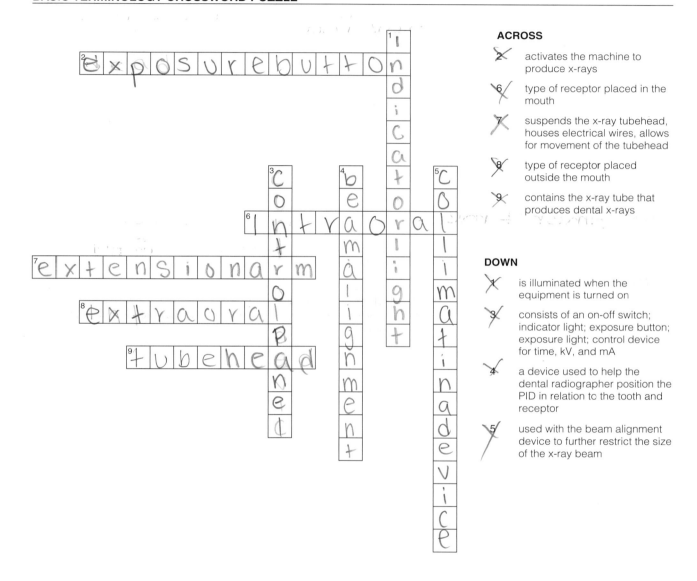

ACROSS

2 activates the machine to produce x-rays

6 type of receptor placed in the mouth

7 suspends the x-ray tubehead, houses electrical wires, allows for movement of the tubehead

8 type of receptor placed outside the mouth

9 contains the x-ray tube that produces dental x-rays

DOWN

1 is illuminated when the equipment is turned on

3 consists of an on-off switch; indicator light; exposure button; exposure light; control device for time, kV, and mA

4 a device used to help the dental radiographer position the PID in relation to the tooth and receptor

5 used with the beam alignment device to further restrict the size of the x-ray beam

Crossword answers:
- 2 ACROSS: exposurebutton
- 6 ACROSS: intraoral
- 7 ACROSS: extensionarm
- 8 ACROSS: extraoral
- 9 ACROSS: tubehead
- 1 DOWN: indicator
- 3 DOWN: controlBpanel
- 4 DOWN: beamalignment
- 5 DOWN: collimatinadevice

Kelsey Rubin

COMPLETION AND SHORT ANSWER

Dental X-Ray Machines

1. List two types of dental x-ray machines: _intraoral_ and _extraoral_.

2. List the functions of each of the following component parts:

   a. Tubehead:

   contains the x-ray that produces dental x-rays, extending from it's the PID

   b. Extension arm:

   Suspends the x-ray tubehead, houses, wires, + allows for movement + position of tubehead

   c. Control panel:

   regulate the x-ray beam include the timer + the kV + mA selectors.

3. No federal standards existed for dental x-ray machines manufactured before the year _1974_.

MULTIPLE CHOICE

Beam Alignment Devices

Circle the correct answer.

1. The anterior RINN device is used on **anterior** / **posterior** teeth.

2. Size **0** / **1** / **2** / **4** receptor is used with the anterior RINN.

3. With the anterior RINN, the receptor is always placed in a **vertical** / **horizontal** direction.

4. The posterior RINN device is used on **anterior** / **posterior** teeth.

5. Size **0** / **1** / **2** / **4** receptor is used with the posterior RINN.

6. With the posterior RINN, the receptor is always placed in a **vertical** / **horizontal** direction.

ACTIVE LEARNING EXPERIENCES

Chapter 6   Dental X-Ray Equipment

IDENTIFICATION AND ASSEMBLY

Anterior RINN

1. Identify parts of the **anterior RINN**; assemble in lab and using the Interactive Exercises on Evolve.

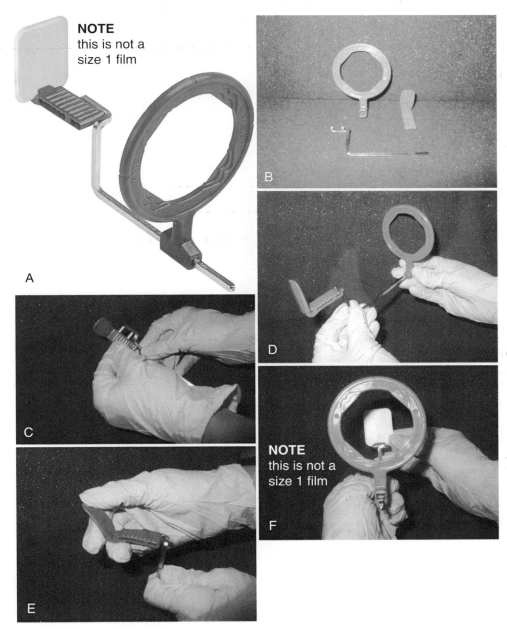

2. After you are comfortable with assembly, work on assembling this RINN as fast as possible.Posterior RINN

1. Identify parts of the **posterior RINN**; assemble in lab and using Interactive Exercises on Evolve.

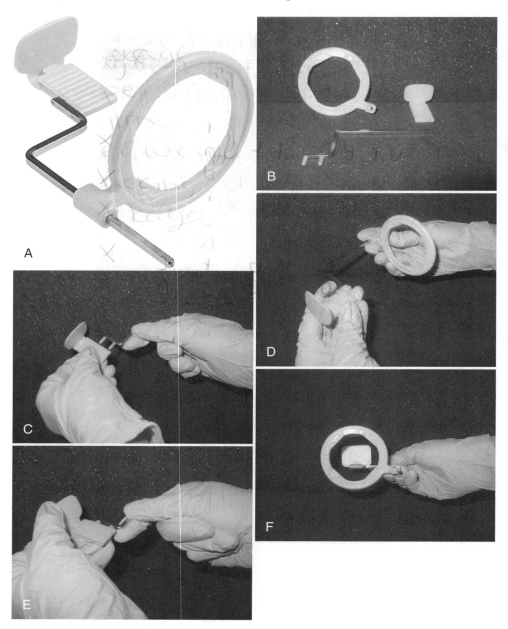

2. After you are comfortable with assembly, work on assembling this RINN as fast as possible.

Bite-Wing RINN

1. Identify parts of the **bite-wing RINN**; assemble in lab and using the Interactive Exercises on Evolve.

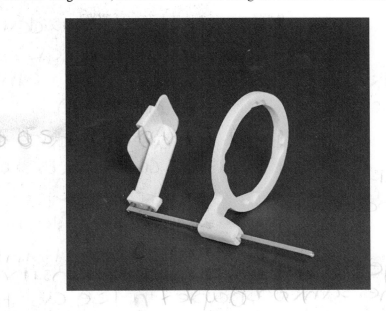

2. After you are comfortable with assembly, work on assembling this RINN as fast as possible.

Module **2** **Equipment, Film, and Processing Basics**

WORKBOOK EXERCISES

Chapter 7   Dental X-Ray Film

BASIC TERMINOLOGY CROSSWORD PUZZLE

ACROSS

6. special type of photographic film used to make a copy of a radiograph; not exposed to x-rays
7. outer side of x-ray film packet that is white and exhibits a raised bump
8. type of intensifying screen that contains phosphors not usually found in the earth
9. something that responds to a stimulus, examples: x-ray film or digital sensors
13. to emit visible light in the blue or green spectrum
14. receptor that consists of a base, adhesive layer, emulsion, and protective layer
15. pattern of stored energy on the exposed film

DOWN

1. type of intensifying screen that contains phosphors that emit blue light
2. light-tight device used to hold film & intensifying screens
3. image that results when a receptor is placed inside the mouth and exposed to x-rays
4. type of screen that converts x-ray energy into visible light
5. extraoral film that is sensitive to the light emitted from intensifying screens
6. small raised bump that appears in one corner of an intraoral film
10. fastest intraoral film available
11. image that results when a receptor is placed outside the mouth and exposed to x-rays
12. outer side of the x-ray film packet that is color coded

Crossword answers:

1 DOWN: calciumtungstate
2 DOWN: cassette
3 DOWN: intraoral
4 DOWN: intensifying
5 DOWN: screen
6 ACROSS: duplicating
7 ACROSS: tubeside
8 ACROSS: rareearth
9 ACROSS: receptor
10 DOWN: fspeed
11 DOWN: extraoral
12 DOWN: labelside
13 ACROSS: fluoresce
14 ACROSS: x-rayfilm
15 ACROSS: latentimage

IDENTIFICATION AND LABELING

Intraoral Film Packet

Identify each item in Fig. 7-1.

1. Outer package
2. inner paper
3. dental film
4. inner paper wrap
5. lead foil backing
6. outer package

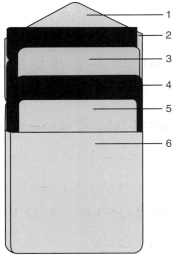

Fig. 7-1

Identify each item in Fig. 7-2.

1. dot on label side of film packet
2. outer package wrapping
3. lead foil sheet
4. black paper film wrapper
5. id dot on tube side
6. intraoral film
7. outer package wrapping

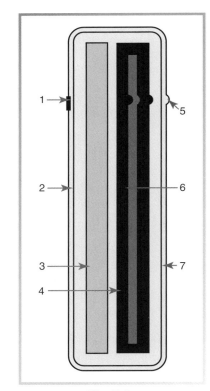

Fig. 7-2

Module **2** **Equipment, Film, and Processing Basics**

Name Kelsey Rubin

Date ___________

Cassette and Screen Film

Identify each item in Fig. 7-3.

1. Front screen
2. Screen film
3. Black screen
4. plastic cassette front
5. screen base
6. phosphor coating
7. screen film
8. phosphor coating
9. screen base
10. metal cassette back

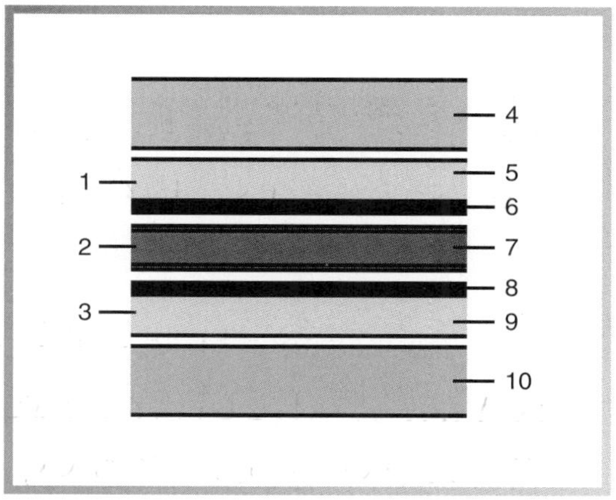

Fig. 7-3

Name Kelsey Rubin
Date 9-30-20

WORKBOOK EXERCISES

Chapter 8 Dental X-Ray Image Characteristics

BASIC TERMINOLOGY CROSSWORD PUZZLE

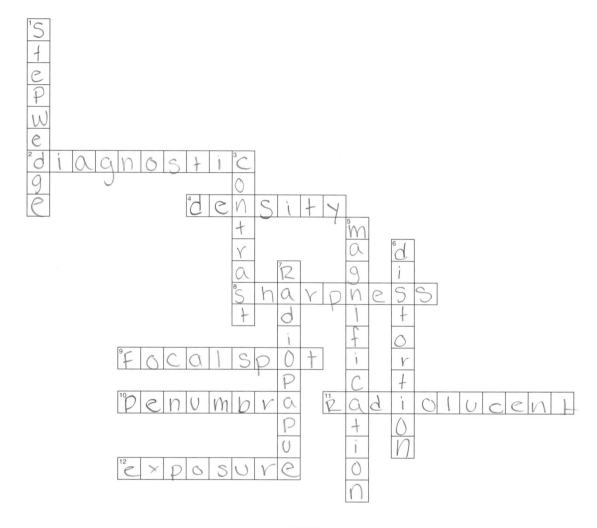

Crossword answers:
- 1 (down) S t e p w e d g e
- 2 (across) d i a g n o s t i c
- 3 (down) c o n t r a s t
- 4 (across) d e n s i t y
- 5 (down) m a g n i f i c a t i o n
- 6 (down) d i s t o r t i o n
- 7 (down) R a d i o p a q u e
- 8 (across) s h a r p n e s s
- 9 (across) F o c a l s p o t
- 10 (across) p e n u m b r a
- 11 (across) R a d i o l u c e n t
- 12 (across) e x p o s u r e

ACROSS

2. image that has proper density and contrast, sharp outlines, and is the same shape and size as the object

4. the overall darkness or blackness of an image

8. refers to the capability of the receptor to reproduce the distinct outlines of an object; influenced by focal spot size, film composition, and movement tungsten

9. target of the anode; converts bombarding electrons into x-ray photons, concentrating the electrons and creating an enormous amount of heat

10. fuzzy, unclear area that surrounds the outline of an image

11. portion of an image that is dark or black

12. a factor that influences the density of an image (mA, kV, exposure time)

DOWN

1. device used to demonstrate film densities and contrast scales

3. how sharply dark and light areas are differentiated or separated on an image

5. geometric characteristic influenced by target-receptor distance and object-receptor distance

6. geometric characteristic that is influenced by object-receptor alignment and x-ray beam angulation

7. portion of an image that is light or white

Kelsey Rubin
9-30-20

Dental X-Ray Image Characteristics

1. Define radiolucent. *Portion of an image that is dark or black, a structure that appears lacks density + permits the passage of x-ray beam with little or no resistance*

2. List one example of what appears radiolucent on a dental image. *air space*

3. Define radiopaque. *Portion of image that appears light or white, structures are dense + absorb or resist the passage of x-ray beam*

4. List one example of what appears radiopaque on a dental image. *enamel, dentin, and bone*

5. Describe a diagnostic image. *provides great deal of information, that images exhibit proper density + contrast are of the same shape + size as the object exposed, and have sharp outlines.*

Visual Characteristics

List the two visual characteristics of the radiographic image.

1. *Contrast*
2. *Density*

Circle the correct answers.

3.	HIGH KV	electron energy is	(high) / low
4.	LOW KV	electron energy is	high / (low)
5.	HIGH MA	electron quantity is	(high) / low
6.	LOW MA	electron quantity is	high / (low)
7.	HIGH KV + MA	image appears	(dark) / light
8.	LOW KV + MA	image appears	dark / (light)
9.	DENSITY	is influenced by	(kV) (mA) / (time)
10.	CONTRAST	is influenced by	(kV) / mA / time
11.	SMALL PATIENT	kV, mA, time must be	increased / (decreased)
12.	LARGE PATIENT	kV, mA, time must be	(increased) / decreased
13.	SHORT SCALE	contrast results from	(low kV) / high kV
14.	LONG SCALE	contrast results from	low kV / (high kV)
15.	HIGH CONTRAST	contrast scale that is	long / (short)
16.	LOW CONTRAST	contrast scale that is	(long) / short

Name Kelsey Rubin
Date 9-30-20

Geometric Characteristics

1. Using the diagram in Fig. 8-1, describe how the size of the focal spot affects the **sharpness** of an image.

When there is a smaller focal spot sharpness is better, and the larger the focal spot the less sharp the image will be.

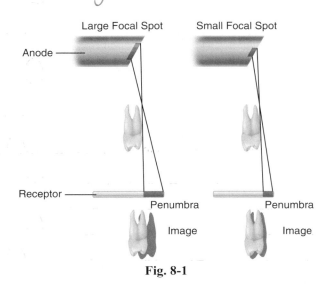

Fig. 8-1

2. Using the diagram in Fig. 8-2, describe how the position indicating device (PID) length affects the **magnification** of an image.

The PID + target receptor distance results in less image magnification

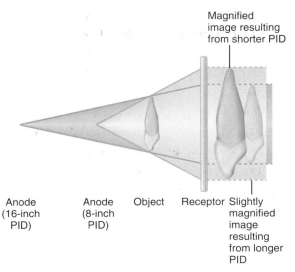

Fig. 8-2

Module **2** **Equipment, Film, and Processing Basics**

Kelsey Rubin
9-30-20

Influencing Factors and Geometric Characteristics

For items 1 to 8, circle ⇧ (increase) or ⇩ (decrease) for each of the following:

Geometric characteristic	Influencing factors	Effects of influencing factors		
Sharpness	Focal spot size	**1** ↓ Focal spot size	(⇧) ⇩	sharpness
		2 ↑ Focal spot size	⇧ (⇩)	sharpness
	Movement	**3** ↓ Movement	(⇧) ⇩	sharpness
		4 ↑ Movement	⇧ (⇩)	sharpness
Magnification	Target-receptor distance	**5** ↑ Target-receptor distance	⇧ (⇩)	magnification
		6 ↓ Target-receptor distance	(⇧) ⇩	magnification
	Object-receptor distance	**7** ↑ Object-receptor distance	(⇧) ⇩	magnification
		8 ↓ Object-receptor distance	⇧ (⇩)	magnification

ACTIVE LEARNING EXPERIENCES

SHADOW CASTING ACTIVITY 1 – SHARPNESS

FOCAL SPOT SIZE

Items Needed

- flashlight   *as large focal spot*

- penlight   *as small focal spot*

- paper cups (3)   *as teeth*

- paper*   *as receptor (*paper in plastic sign holder 8 ½" × 11")*

- tape measure

Concept

- **What?** Focal spot should be as **SMALL** as possible.

- **Why?** To create a **SHARP** image.

Demonstration

- penlight *(small focal spot)* creates a SHARPER shadow

- flashlight *(larger focal spot)* creates a LESS SHARP shadow

Reminders

- the **SMALLER** the focal spot, the **SHARPER** the image

- actual focal spot size in x-ray machine is 0.6-1.0 mm^2

To Do

- In a darkened room, place three cups in a row, touching.

- Place the sign holder 2" behind and parallel to the cups.

- Place the **flashlight** 8" from the cups and direct the beam perpendicular (┬) to the cups. Note the shadow.

- Keep the cups and sign holder in same position and change to the **penlight.**

- Place the **penlight** 8" from the cups and direct the beam perpendicular (┬) to the cups. Note the shadow.

55

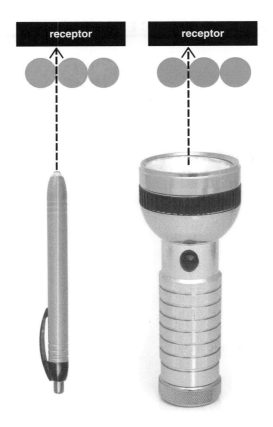

Questions

1. Which creates a smaller shadow—the flashlight or penlight? _____

   _____

2. How does this relate to **focal spot size**?

   _____

   _____

SHADOW CASTING ACTIVITY 2 – MAGNIFICATION

TARGET-RECEPTOR DISTANCE

Items Needed

- flashlight   *as target*

- paper cups (3)   *as teeth*

- paper*   *as receptor (*paper in plastic sign holder 8 ½" × 11")*

- tape measure

Concept

- **What? Target-receptor distance** should be as **LONG** as possible.

- **Why?** To **LIMIT** magnification.

Demonstration

- flashlight at 16″   creates SMALLEST shadow

- flashlight at 12″   creates LARGER shadow

- flashlight at 8″   creates LARGEST shadow

Reminders

- **LONGER** distance   results in **LESS** magnification

- 16″ distance   creates less magnification than 12″

- 12″ distance   creates less magnification than 8″

To Do

- Place cups and sign holder in same position as described in Activity 1.

- For each distance listed below, direct the beam perpendicular (⊥) to the cups.

- Place the flashlight **8″** from the cups. Note the shadow.

- Place the flashlight **12″** from the cups. Note the shadow.

- Place the flashlight **16″** from the cups. Note the shadow.

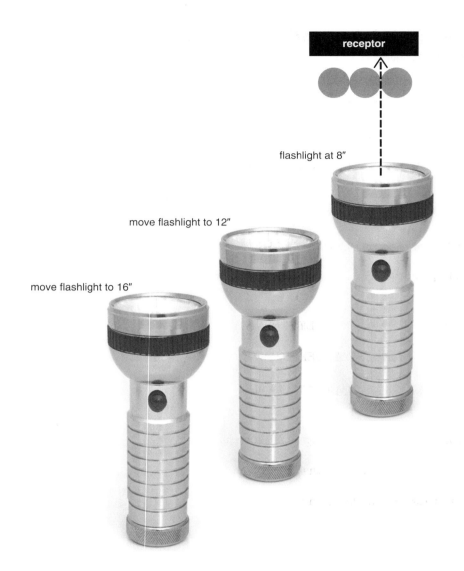

receptor

flashlight at 8″

move flashlight to 12″

move flashlight to 16″

Questions

1. Which distance creates the smallest shadow? _____

2. How does this relate to PID length and **target-receptor distance**?

_____

_____

SHADOW CASTING ACTIVITY 3 – MAGNIFICATION

OBJECT-RECEPTOR DISTANCE

Items Needed

- flashlight   *as target*

- paper cups (3)   *as teeth (object)*

- paper*   *as receptor (*paper in plastic sign holder 8 ½" × 11")*

- tape measure

Concept

- **What? Object-receptor distance** should be as **CLOSE** as possible.

- **Why?** To limit magnification.

Demonstration

- object 0" from receptor   creates SMALLEST shadow

- object 4" from receptor   creates LARGER shadow

- object 8" from receptor   creates LARGEST shadow

Reminders

- if object is **CLOSE** to receptor, **LESS** magnification results

- 0" distance creates less magnification than 4"

- 4" distance creates less magnification than 8"

To Do

- Place the flashlight **8"** from the cups.

- For each distance listed below, direct the beam perpendicular (⊥) to the cups.

- Place the sign holder parallel to and **0"** from the cups. Note the shadow.

- Place the sign holder parallel to and **4"** from the cups. Note the shadow.

- Place the sign holder parallel to and **8"** from the cups. Note the shadow.

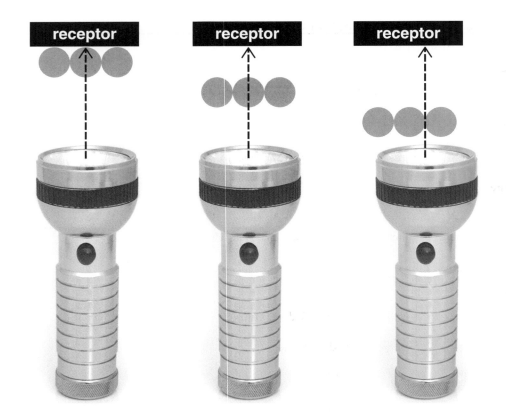

Questions

1. Which shadow is smallest? _____

2. How does this relate to **object-receptor distance**?

_____

_____

SHADOW CASTING ACTIVITY 4 – DISTORTION

OBJECT-RECEPTOR ORIENTATION

Items Needed

- flashlight   *as target*

- paper cups (3)   *as teeth (object)*

- paper*   *as receptor (*paper in plastic sign holder 8 ½" × 11")*

- tape measure

Concept

- **What?** Object and receptor must be **PARALLEL.**

- **Why?** To **LIMIT** distortion.

Demonstration

- object PARALLEL with receptor creates LEAST distortion

- object NOT parallel with receptor creates distortion

- shadow CLOSEST to teeth appears SMALL

- shadow FARTHEST from teeth appears LARGE

Reminders

- object and receptor should be **PARALLEL** to limit distortion

To Do

- Place the flashlight 16" from the cups.

- Place the sign holder parallel to and 8" from the cups Note the shadow.

- Place the sign holder NOT parallel to and 8" from the cups. Note the shadow.

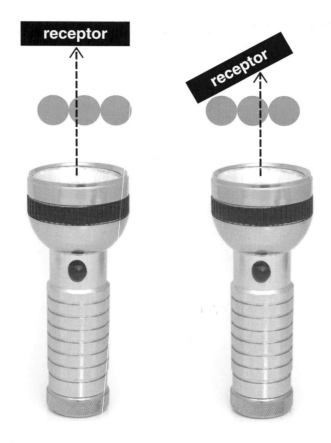

Questions

1. How does the shadow change? _____
   _____

2. How does the shadow appear on parts of the sign holder **closest** to the cups?
   _____
   _____

3. How does the shadow appear on parts of the sign holder **farthest** from the cups?
   _____
   _____

4. How does this relate to **distortion**?
   _____
   _____

SHADOW CASTING ACTIVITY 5 – DISTORTION

ELONGATED AND FORESHORTENED IMAGES

Items Needed

- flashlight   *as target*

- paper cups (3)   *as teeth (object)*

- paper*   *as receptor (*paper in plastic sign holder 8 ½" × 11")*

- tape measure

Concept

- **What? Correct beam angulation** creates an image that resembles the object.

- **Why?** To **LIMIT** distortion.

Demonstration

- **STEEP** beam angulation   shadow is **SHORT** (foreshortened)

- **FLAT** beam angulation   shadow is **LONG** (elongated)

To Do

- Place the sign holder against the bottom of the cups and then tip it 3" from the top of the cups.

- Angle the flashlight, direct the beam down at a **+ 70°** angle to the table. Note the shadow.

- Angle the flashlight, direct the beam down at a **+ 20°** angle to the table. Note the shadow.

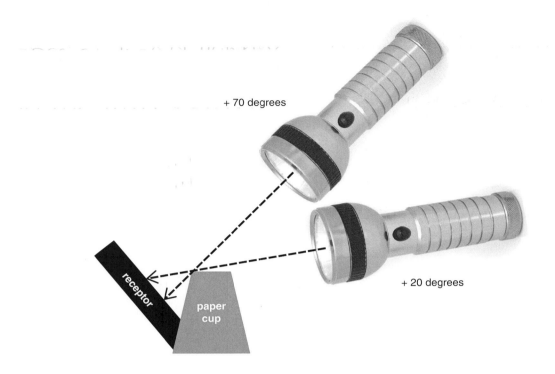

+ 70 degrees

+ 20 degrees

receptor

paper
cup

Questions

1. What happens when the vertical angulation is steep (+70°)? Is the shadow shorter or longer?

_____

2. What happens when the vertical angulation is flat (+20°)? Is the shadow shorter or longer?

_____

3. How does this relate to **distortion**?

_____

_____

WORKBOOK EXERCISES

Chapter 9   Film Processing

BASIC TERMINOLOGY CROSSWORD PUZZLE

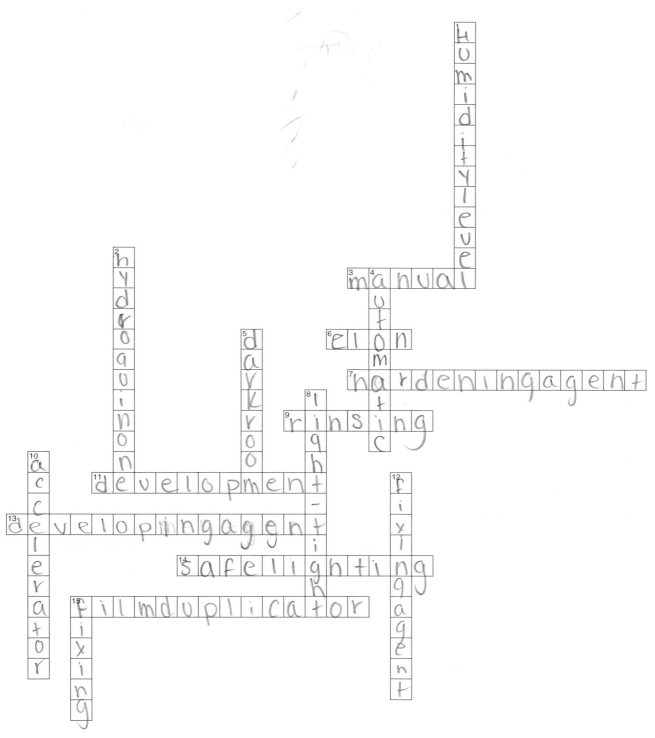

Crossword solution:
- 1 Down: humiditylevel
- 2 Down: hydroquinon
- 3 Across: manual
- 4 Down: automatic
- 5 Down: darkroom
- 6 Across: elon
- 7 Across: hardeningagent
- 8 Down: light-tight
- 9 Across: rinsing
- 10 Down: accelerator
- 11 Across: development
- 12 Down: fixingagent
- 13 Across: developingagent
- 14 Across: safelighting
- 15 Across: filmduplicator
- 15 Down: fixing

ACROSS

3   a type of processing where all steps are performed manually

6   chemical found in the developing agent that generates the many shades of gray of the radiographic image

7   a basic ingredient of the fixer solution; contains the chemical potassium alum, which hardens and shrinks the gelatin in the film emulsion

9   one of the five steps in film processing; a water bath is used to remove the developer from the film and stop the development process

11   first step in film processing; the developer solution reduces the halides in the film emulsion to black metallic silver and softens the film emulsion

13   a basic ingredient of the developer; contains two chemicals, hydroquinone and elon, which reduce halides in the film emulsion to black metallic silver

14   in a darkroom, a low-intensity light composed of long wavelengths in the red-orange portion of the visible light spectrum

15   a light source used to expose duplicating film

DOWN

1   the amount of moisture in the air

2   chemical found in the developing agent that generates the black tones and sharp contrast of the radiographic image

4   a type of film processing where all film processing steps are automated

5   a completely darkened room where x-ray film is handled and processed

8   term used to describe the darkroom, a room that is completely dark and excludes all white light

10   a basic ingredient of the developer; sodium carbonate activates and provides an alkaline environment for the developing agents and softens the film emulsion

12   a basic ingredient of the fixer solution; contains hypo, which removes or clears all unexposed and undeveloped silver halide crystals from the film emulsion

15   step in film processing; removes the unexposed, undeveloped silver halide crystals from the film emulsion and hardens the film emulsion

IDENTIFICATION AND LABELING

Automatic Processor

Identify the components in Fig. 9-1.

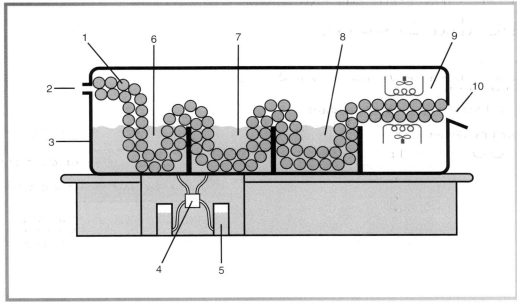

Fig. 9-1

1. Roller film transporter
2. Film feed slot
3. Processor housing
4. Replenisher pump
5. Replenisher solutions
6. Developer compartment
7. Fixer compartment
8. Water compartment
9. Drying chamber
10. Film recovery slot

Kelsey Rubin

Safelighting

1. Describe safelighting.

   Special type of lighting
   used to provide illumination
   in the darkroom

2. Explain why the 4-foot distance is important.

   films that are unwrapped
   too close will appear
   fogged

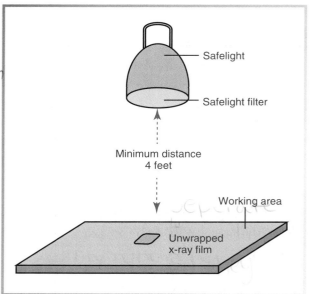

Safelight

Safelight filter

Minimum distance
4 feet

Working area

Unwrapped
x-ray film

Name Kelsey Rubin
Date 9-24

MULTIPLE CHOICE, SHORT ANSWER AND IDENTIFICATION

For numbers 1 to 22 below, circle the correct answer choice or fill in the missing information.

Time and Temperature Problems

ERROR	APPEARANCE	PROBLEM	SOLUTION
	light	1. Development time is ~~too short~~ / too long.	Check development time.
		2. Developer solution is ~~too cool~~ / too warm.	Check developer temperature.
		3. Developer solution ~~too weak~~ / too strong.	Replenish developer with fresh solution as needed.
	dark	4. Development time is too short / ~~too long.~~	Check development time.
		5. Developer solution is too cool / ~~too warm.~~	Check developer temperature.
		6. Developer solution is too weak / ~~too strong.~~	Replenish developer with fresh solution as needed.
7. Identify error: unsure	cracked	Sudden temperature change between developer and water bath.	Check temperature of processing solutions and water bath; avoid drastic temperature differences.

Chemical Contamination Problems

ERROR	APPEARANCE	PROBLEM	SOLUTION
Developer spots	8. Spots are ~~dark~~ ~~(black)~~ / white (light).	Developer contacts film before processing.	Use a clean work area in the darkroom.
Fixer spots	9. Spots are dark (black) / ~~white (light).~~	Fixer contacts film before processing.	Use a clean work area in the darkroom.
Yellow-brown color	Yellow-brown color	Exhausted developer or fixer	Replenish chemicals with fresh solutions as needed.
		10. Fixing time is ~~too long~~ / too short.	Use adequate fixing time.
		11. Rinsing time is ~~too long~~ / too short.	Rinse for a minimum of 20 minutes.

Module 2 Equipment, Film, and Processing Basics

Kelsey Rubin

Film-Handling Problems

ERROR	APPEARANCE	PROBLEM	SOLUTION
Developer cutoff	12. A straight border that is (white /) black	Undeveloped portion of film due to low level of developer	Check developer level before processing; add solution if needed.
Fixer cutoff	13. A straight border that is (white /) black	Unfixed portion of film due to low level of fixer	Check fixer level before processing; add solution if needed.
	White or dark areas appear on film where overlapped	Two films contacting each other during processing	14. Describe solution: _Seperate the films so they don't overlap._
Air bubbles	White spots	Air trapped on the film surface after being placed in the processing solutions	Gently agitate film racks after placing in processing solutions.
	Black, crescent-shaped marks	Film emulsion damaged by operator's fingernail during rough handling	15. Describe solution: _handle with care, don't put finger nail on film._
	Black fingerprint	Film touched by fingers contaminated with fluoride or developer	16. Describe solution: _make sure to wash + dry hands before handeling_
17. Identify error: _scratching films_	Thin, black, branching lines	Occurs when a film packet is opened quickly and before operator touches a conductive object	18. Describe solution: _open packet slowly_

Name _Kelsey Rubin_

Date _9-24_

ERROR	APPEARANCE	PROBLEM	SOLUTION
19. Identify error: scratched film	White lines	Soft emulsion removed from film by a sharp object	Use care when handling films and film racks.

Lighting Problems

ERROR	APPEARANCE	PROBLEM	SOLUTION
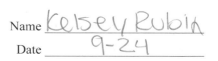	Exposed area appears black	Accidental exposure of film to white light	**20. Describe solution:** inspect film packet before using
21. Identify error: fogging film	Gray; lacks detail and contrast	Improper safelighting Light leaks in darkroom Outdated films Improper film storage Contaminated solutions **22.** Developer solution **too cool** / **too warm** (circled)	Check filter and bulb wattage of safelight. Check darkroom for light leaks. Check the expiration date on film packages. Store films in a cool, dry, and protected area. Avoid contaminated solutions by covering tanks after use. Check temperature of developer.

Module **2** Equipment, Film, and Processing Basics

WORKBOOK EXERCISES

Chapter 10   Quality Assurance

BASIC TERMINOLOGY CROSSWORD PUZZLE

ACROSS

6. specific tests designed to maintain and monitor dental x-ray equipment, supplies, and film processing

DOWN

1. the management of the quality assurance plan in the dental office

2. a radiograph processed under ideal conditions and then used to compare the film densities of radiographs that are processed daily

3. commercially available device used to monitor developer strength and film density

4. a light source used to view dental radiographs (also called the illuminator)

5. a device constructed of uniform-layered thicknesses of an x-ray absorbing material, usually aluminum; different steps absorb varying amounts of x-rays and are used to demonstrate film densities and contrast scales

6. special procedures used to ensure the production of high-quality diagnostic images

Crossword answers filled in:

- 1 Down: quality administration
- 2 Down: reference
- 3 Down: normalizing
- 4 Down: viewbox
- 5 Down: stepwedge
- 6 Across: quality control tests
- 6 Down: quality assurance

Kelsey Rubin
9-24

IDENTIFICATION AND SHORT ANSWER

For each test listed, place an **X** in the box that indicates the suggested frequency of testing; if "other" is chosen, add notes to clarify how often.

	Daily	Weekly	Monthly	Yearly	Other	Special notes
DENTAL X-RAY MACHINES						
1. All quality control tests				X		Also: upon installation, inspection by a qualified expert
DENTAL X-RAY FILM						
2. Rotate stock					X	When no box isopened
3. Fresh film test					X	Only when new box is opened
SCREENS AND CASSETTES						
4. Clean			X			
5. Inspect			X			
6. Contact test			X			
DARKROOM						
7. Light leak test			X			
8. Safelight test					X	every 6 months
PROCESSING EQUIPMENT AND SOLUTIONS						
9. Temperature check–solutions	X					
10. Quality control tests	X					
11. Replenish solutions	X					
12. Drain and clean	X					
13. Change solutions	X					
VIEW BOX						
14. Plexiglass surface					X	just said periodically
15. Lightbulbs					X	When blackened
16. Clean		X			X	
DIGITAL IMAGING EQUIPMENT						
17. Computer data backup	X					
18. Digital sensors	X					
19. Imaging plates	X					
20. Wired attachments	X					

MULTIPLE CHOICE

Identify the choice that best completes the statement or answers the question.

1. Extraoral intensifying screens that appear visibly scratched should…

    a. be cleaned with commercially available cleaner.
    b. have antistatic solution applied.
    c. be replaced.
    d. be polished and then reused.

2. To conduct the film-screen contact test, the PID should have a _____-inch target-film distance.

    a. 6
    b. 12
    c. 40
    d. 72

3. Which is true concerning the evaluation of the film-screen contact test?

    a. Areas of poor film-screen contact appear darker than good contact areas.
    b. Areas of poor film-screen contact appear lighter than good contact areas.
    c. If the wire mesh image on the film exhibits varying densities, good film-screen contact has taken place.
    d. Both a and c.

4. During the light-leak test for the darkroom…

    a. a flashlight should be used to check for light leaks.
    b. the overhead lights should be off but the safelight should be on.
    c. all lights within the darkroom should be off.
    d. light a match within the darkroom and see if any light is visible from the outside.

5. To conduct the coin test, the film and coin are exposed for…

    a. 10 seconds.
    b. 3 or 4 minutes.
    c. 15 minutes.
    d. an entire workday.

6. To test the automatic film processor, _____ in the automatic processor.

    a. unwrap one film, expose it to light, and then process the film
    b. unwrap one film, do not expose it to light, and then process the film
    c. unwrap two unexposed films, expose one to light, and then process the exposed film
    d. unwrap two unexposed films, expose one to light, and then process both films

Kelsey Rubin 9-24

7. To create a reference radiograph, which of the following must be fresh?

      I.   Film
     II. Developer
   III. Fixer

  a. I, II, and III
  b. I, II
  c. II, III
  d. I only

8. A reference radiograph is compared with a radiograph taken each day for matched…

  a. milliamperage.
  b. kV.
  c. color.
  d. density.

9. When the stepwedge technique is used to evaluate developer strength, if the density on the daily radiograph differs from that on the standard radiograph by more than _____ steps, the developer solution is depleted.

  a. two
  b. three
  c. five
  d. seven

10. The clearing test is used to monitor…

  a. developer strength.
  b. fixer strength.
  c. water bath temperature.
  d. processing speed.

APPLICATION

Module 2 Equipment, Film, and Processing

SELF-ASSESSMENT

Chapters 6 - 10

Based on the worksheets that you have just completed for Chapters 6 - 10, how prepared are you for assessments?

_____ very prepared, confident

_____ somewhat prepared, somewhat confident

_____ somewhat unprepared, lack confidence

_____ unprepared, no confidence

Based on your answer above, what is your plan for improvement? List the topics and concepts that you need to further review and study for assessments.

_____

_____

_____

_____

_____

_____

CRITICAL THINKING QUESTIONS

What does all of the information in Chapters 6 to 10 mean to you in the practice setting? Use the questions below to help you apply the information that you have just learned. Work in pairs and practice answering these questions with your classmates. Share feedback concerning the content and delivery of information—is the information correct and understandable for the average patient? Are effective communication skills being used? The more you practice, the more comfortable you will be discussing these issues with your patients.

1. A patient calls and states that he is moving to another state and needs his dental images before he moves next week. What should the dental radiographer prepare for the patient?

   • CHAPTER 7

2. You are using a stepwedge film to evaluate the quality of the developer solution. You note that the middle density on the daily film is much lighter than the middle density on the stepwedge film. What is the problem, and how do you solve it?

   • CHAPTER 8

   • CHAPTER 10

3. A new assistant has just been hired and has been instructed to help the dental hygienist with imaging of two new patients. The dental hygienist exposes the first set of images and instructs the new assistant to develop the films while the dental hygienist continues with the second patient. After developing the x-rays the new assistant presents the x-rays to the dental hygienist. The x-rays have a yellow-brown color and are unreadable. How should this situation be handled? Should the x-rays be retaken?

   • CHAPTER 9

4. A new assistant has recently been hired at your office. The automatic processor in your office is under repair, and the repair company did not issue your office a loaner. During your morning routine, you are explaining the situation to the new assistant. At this point, she informs you that she is unfamiliar with processing dental films manually. What should you do to handle this situation properly?

   • CHAPTER 9

5. A new assistant has just been hired and has been instructed to take all of the x-rays for new patients. After she takes her first full-mouth series and develops them, she notices that they all have a straight white border along the edge that cuts off part of the image. How should this situation be handled? Should the x-rays be retaken?

   • CHAPTER 9

6. A dental assistant has just started working at a new office. The staff informs the new assistant that in the past they have had problems with x-rays having to be retaken. The previous dental assistant in charge of quality assurance had trouble finding time to follow up on quality control tests and realized something was wrong only when the staff was busy attending to another patient. What sort of plan should the new dental assistant implement? How can the dental assistant ensure that the plan doesn't interfere with time allocated for patient treatment?

   • CHAPTER 10

TO-DO CHECKLIST

Written Exercises

_____ Complete all worksheets.

_____ Complete self-assessment.

Active Learning Experiences

_____ Identify and assemble RINN devices.

_____ Identify parts of the intraoral film packet, sizes of film, bite-wing tab, extraoral film, intensifying screens, and cassette.

_____ Complete the shadow casting exercises.

_____ Review and answer the critical thinking questions; practice answering them with your classmates and provide feedback.

_____ Review and answer the critical thinking questions.

_____ Practice answering critical thinking questions with your classmates and provide feedback.

Clinical Laboratory Activities

_____ Complete activities in Section 2, _Laboratory Manual_, Part 1 - Introduction to the Radiology Clinic _(as assigned by instructor)._

Assessments

_____ Complete assessments in Section 2, _Laboratory Manual_, Part 1 - Introduction to the Radiology Clinic _(as assigned by instructor)._

RINN ASSEMBLY REVIEW

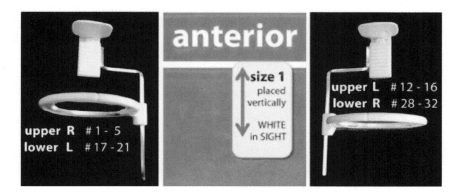

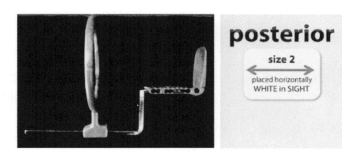

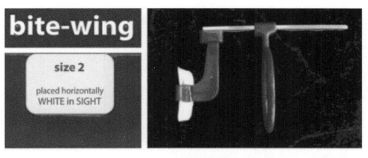

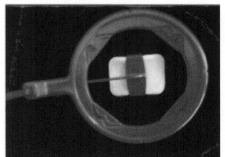

FILM SIZE SUMMARY

Size **0**

22 × 35 mm
or
7/8 in ×
1 3/8 in

Size 0
used in small children
periapical or **bite-wing**

Size **1**

24 × 40 mm
or
15/16 in × 1 9/16 in

Size 1
periapicals (anterior)

Size **2**

30.5 × 40.5 mm
or
1 1/4 in × 1 5/8 in

Size 2
periapicals (anterior or
posterior) or **bite-wings**

Size **4**

57 × 76 mm
or
2 1/4 in × 3 in

Size 4
occlusal

82

RADIOLUCENT

- air space
- foramen
- canal
- suture
- fossa
- pdl space

- soft tissue

- cancellous bone

- cortical bone
- lamina dura
- dentin
- enamel

- metal restorations

RADIOPAQUE

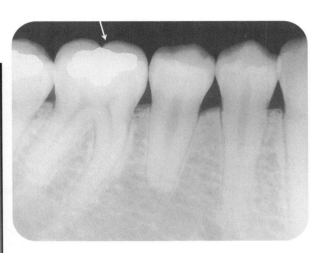

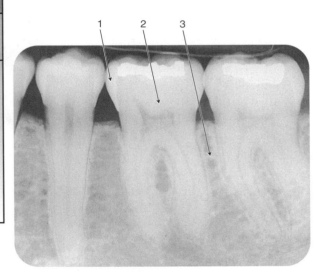

ELONGATION AND FORESHORTENING REVIEW

The incorrect vertical angulation of the PID will distort the image and result in *elongation* or *foreshortening*.

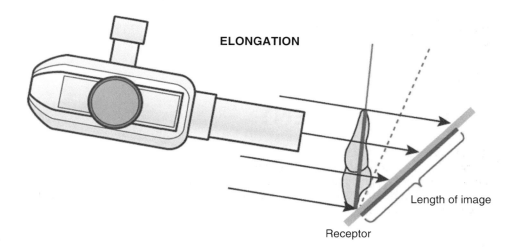

ELONGATION

Length of image

Receptor

In ELONGATION:
- The PID is too **FLAT**.
- **LONG** image
- To correct this, you must **increase** the PID angle.
- Compare the length of the **image** to the length of the **tooth**.
- The image appears **LONG** (stretched).
  Too **FLAT**
  Too **LONG**

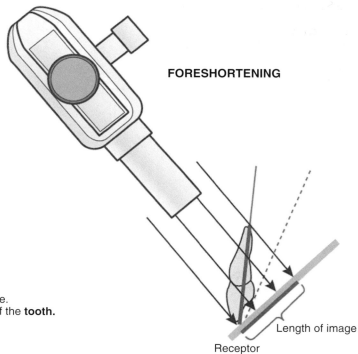

FORESHORTENING

In FORESHORTENING:
- The PID is too **STEEP**.
- **SHORT** image
- To correct this, you must **decrease** the PID angle.
- Compare the length of the **image** to the length of the **tooth**.
- The image appears **SHORT**.
  Too **STEEP**
  Too **SHORT**

Length of image

Receptor

INSTRUCTIONS

How to Prepare
- Review the learning objectives for Module 3 prior to lab.
- Review the critical thinking questions for Module 3 prior to lab.

What to Bring
- *Workbook and Laboratory Manual*—Module 3 materials
- pencil
- textbook (print or e-version)
- typodont

Written Exercises
- Work together or individually to complete each exercise.
- For each chapter, complete the worksheets in pencil (*without looking up answers*).
- When each exercise is finished, use your text to check answers; correct any wrong answers.
- Use your completed and corrected packet to study for assessments.

Active Learning Experiences
- Practice assembly of RINN devices.
- Practice film placements utilizing the paralleling technique on a typodont.
- In pairs, take turns answering each critical thinking question and provide feedback to each other.
- Ask your instructor to observe you answering the critical thinking questions and provide you with feedback.

Clinical Laboratory Activities
- See Section 2, *Laboratory Manual*.

Assessments
- See Section 2, *Laboratory Manual*.

3 Radiographer and Technique Basics

LEARNING OBJECTIVES

The goal of Module 3 laboratory experiences is to provide students with a reinforcement of the fundamental understanding of radiographer and technique basics. Upon successful completion of Chapters 11 to 17 lectures and laboratory, the student will be able to:

CHAPTER	LEARNING OBJECTIVES
CHAPTER 11 DENTAL IMAGES AND THE DENTAL RADIOGRAPHER	
Written Exercises	• Summarize the importance and use of dental images. • List your professional goals for becoming a competent radiographer.
CHAPTER 12 PATIENT RELATIONS AND THE DENTAL RADIOGRAPHER	
Written Exercises	• Recognize words used in dentistry that are associated with negative images. • Describe the ideal chairside manner and attitude of the dental radiographer.
CHAPTER 13 PATIENT EDUCATION AND THE DENTAL RADIOGRAPHER	
Written Exercises	• Answer common patient questions about dental x-rays. • Summarize the importance of educating patients about dental x-rays.
CHAPTER 14 LEGAL ISSUES AND THE DENTAL RADIOGRAPHER	
Written Exercises	• Define basic terminology used with legal issues and dental imaging. • Review ownership, retention, and refusal of dental images.
CHAPTER 15 INFECTION CONTROL AND THE DENTAL RADIOGRAPHER	
Written Exercises	• Define basic terminology used with infection control. • Describe receptor handling and infection control used in dental imaging.
CHAPTER 16 INTRODUCTION TO DENTAL IMAGING EXAMINATIONS	
Written Exercises	• Define basic terminology used with dental imaging examinations. • Apply guidelines for prescribing dental images to typical patient encounters.
CHAPTER 17 PARALLELING TECHNIQUE	
Written Exercises	• Identify basic concepts of the paralleling technique. • Draw periapical receptor placements and identify proper exposure technique. • Complete periapical assessment exercises. • Define basic terminology used with the paralleling technique. • Assemble RINN devices, demonstrate placement of receptors in RINN devices, and demonstrate positioning of the RINN device on a typodont.

MODULE 3 CLINICAL LABORATORY ACTIVITIES

• Apply information learned to complete activities in Section 2, *Laboratory Manual (as assigned by instructor).*

MODULE 3 ASSESSMENTS

• Apply information learned to complete assessments in Section 2, *Laboratory Manual (as assigned by instructor).*

WORKBOOK EXERCISES

Chapter 11   Dental Images and the Dental Radiographer

SHORT ANSWER

Dental Images

1. Briefly summarize the importance and uses of dental images.

   _____

   _____

   _____

   _____

   _____

Dental Radiographer

Describe your commitment to each of the following professional goals:

1. Patient protection: _____

   _____

   _____

2. Operator protection: _____

   _____

   _____

3. Patient education: _____

   _____

   _____

4. Operator competence: _____

   _____

   _____

5. Operator efficiency: _____

   _____

   _____

6. Production of quality images: _____

   _____

   _____

WORKBOOK EXERCISES

Chapter 12 Patient Relations and the Dental Radiographer

IDENTIFICATION

Communication Skills

For each of the following, place an **X** next to words that are associated with negative images in the dental setting.

1. _____ restore

2. _____ cut

3. _____ pain

4. _____ discomfort

5. _____ drill

6. _____ scrape

7. _____ zap

8. _____ hurt

9. _____ false teeth

10. _____ waiting room

For each of the following, place an **X** next to appropriate communication messages.

11. _____ checking the time on your watch while the patient is talking

12. _____ nodding head to indicate agreement with the patient

13. _____ using direct eye contact while listening to patient

14. _____ folding arms across chest while listening to patient

15. _____ leaning slightly toward the patient while talking

16. _____ interrupting the patient to save time

17. _____ conducting personal conversations with other staff in earshot of patient

18. _____ rolling eyes when a staff member leaves the area

19. _____ finishing the patient's sentences to keep patient on track

SHORT ANSWER

Communication Skills

Briefly describe why each of the following phrases should be avoided in the dental setting.

1. "Sorry 'bout that." _____

_____

_____

2. "Just relax." _____

_____

_____

3. "Calm down." _____

_____

_____

4. "I don't know." _____

_____

_____

5. "Not a problem." _____

_____

_____

6. "It's crazy around here today." _____

_____

_____

Chairside Manner and Patient Relations

1. Briefly describe the chairside manner that is appropriate in the dental setting. _____

_____

_____

2. Briefly describe the attitude that is appropriate in the dental setting. _____

_____

_____

Name _____

Date _____

WORKBOOK EXERCISES

Chapter 13 Patient Education and the Dental Radiographer

SHORT ANSWER

Importance of Patient Education

1. Briefly describe the importance of patient education concerning x-rays. _____

_____

_____

Common Questions and Answers

Answer each of these questions as detailed in Chapter 13 of the text.

1. Are dental x-ray images really necessary? _____

_____

_____

_____

_____

2. How often do I need dental x-ray images? _____

_____

_____

_____

_____

3. Can I refuse x-rays and be treated without the images? _____

_____

_____

_____

_____

4. Can you use the dental x-ray images from my previous dentist? _____

_____

_____

_____

_____

5. How do you limit my exposure to x-rays? _____

_____

_____

_____

_____

6. Why do you use a lead apron? _____

_____

_____

_____

_____

7. Should I avoid dental x-ray exposure during pregnancy? _____

_____

_____

_____

_____

8. Why do you leave the room when x-rays are used? _____

_____

_____

_____

_____

9. Are dental x-rays safe? _____

_____

_____

_____

_____

10. Will dental x-ray exposure cause cancer? _____

_____

_____

_____

_____

11. What are the advantages to using digital imaging? _____

_____

_____

_____

_____

12. Are there risks associated with digital imaging? _____

_____

_____

_____

_____

12. Who owns my dental x-ray images? _____

_____

_____

_____

_____

WORKBOOK EXERCISES

Chapter 14   Legal Issues and the Dental Radiographer

BASIC TERMINOLOGY CROSSWORD PUZZLE

ACROSS

10   period during which a patient may bring a malpractice action against a dentist or an auxiliary

DOWN

1   legal rights of an individual to make choices about the care he or she receives, including the opportunity to consent to or refuse treatment

2   permission given by a patient following complete disclosure about the particulars of a procedure

3   private; in dental imaging, information contained in the dental record is _____

4   improper or negligent conduct or treatment

5   legal accountability

6   in dental imaging, the process of informing a patient about the particulars of exposing dental images

7   policies and procedures that the dental professional should follow to reduce the chance that a patient will take legal action against the dental professional or the supervising dentist

8   omission or failure to provide reasonable precaution, care, or action; occurs when the diagnosis made or the dental treatment delivered falls below the standard of care

9   in dentistry, the quality of care that is provided by dental practitioners in a similar locality under the same or similar conditions

SHORT ANSWER

Legal Issues and the Dental Patient

1. Briefly discuss the ownership and retention of dental images. _____

_____

_____

_____

_____

2. Briefly discuss patients who refuse dental images. _____

_____

_____

_____

_____

3. List the four essential elements of informed consent.

a. _____

b. _____

c. _____

d. _____

4. In regards to dental imaging, list the four essential elements of documentation.

a. _____

b. _____

c. _____

d. _____

TRUE OR FALSE

Legal Issues and the Dental Patient

1. _____ Dental images are the property of the patient.

2. _____ Dental records should be retained indefinitely.

3. _____ A patient has reasonable access to his or her dental record.

4. _____ A dentist may release a patient's original images and retain a copy for office records.

5. _____ The dental record, including images, is a legal document.

6. _____ All images in the dental record are confidential.

WORKBOOK EXERCISES

Chapter 15   Infection Control and the Dental Radiographer

BASIC TERMINOLOGY CROSSWORD PUZZLE

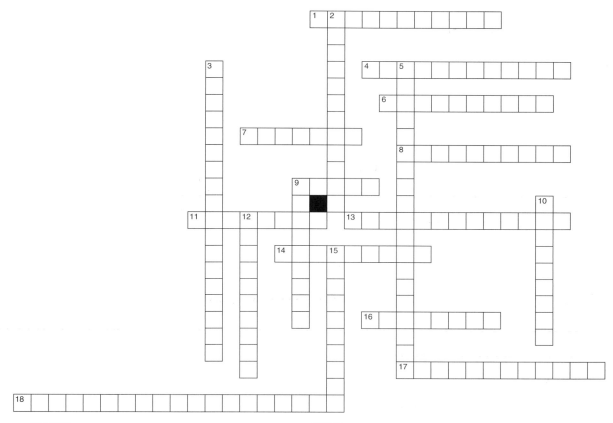

ACROSS

1   category of instruments that do not come in contact with mucous membranes

4   the act of disinfecting

6   type of exposure/contact with blood or other infectious materials that results from piercing or puncturing the skin barrier

7   absence of pathogens or disease-causing microorganisms

8   substance that inhibits the growth of bacteria

9   any object that can penetrate skin, including, but not limited to, needles and scalpels

11   a microorganism capable of causing disease

13   the act of sterilizing

14   to inhibit or destroy disease-causing microorganisms through use of a chemical or physical procedure

16   category of instruments that are used to penetrate soft tissue or bone; must be sterilized after each use

17   category of instruments that contact but do not penetrate soft tissue or bone; must be sterilized after each use

18   microorganisms present in blood that cause disease in humans

DOWN

2   type of exposure/contact with blood or other infectious materials involving the skin, eye, or mucous membranes that results from procedures performed by the dental professional

3   a category of disinfectant classified by the EPA as both "hospital disinfectants" and "tuberculocidals"; recommended for all surfaces that have been contaminated

5   standard of care designed to protect health care personnel and patients from pathogens, blood, or any other body fluid, excretion, or secretion

9   the use of a physical or chemical procedure to destroy all pathogens, including highly resistant bacterial and fungal spores

10   a category of disinfectant classified by the EPA as "hospital disinfectants"; recommended for general housekeeping purposes

12   a category of disinfectant classified by the EPA as "sterilants-disinfectants"; used to disinfect heat-sensitive, semicritical dental instruments

15   type of waste that consists of blood, blood products, contaminated sharps, or other microbiologic products

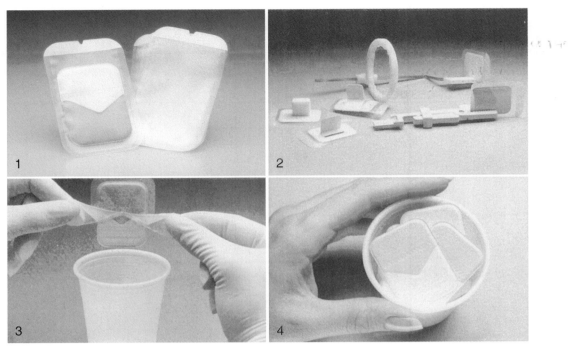

Fig. 15-1

IDENTIFY AND DESCRIBE

Infection Control Procedures

For each photo in Fig. 15-1, describe what you see as it pertains to infection control in dental imaging.

1. _____

_____

_____

2. _____

_____

_____

3. _____

_____

_____

4. _____

_____

_____

SHORT ANSWER

Infection Control Procedures

1. List the five indications for hand hygiene.

   a. _____

   b. _____

   c. _____

   d. _____

   e. _____

2. List the three types of hand hygiene that may be used in dental imaging.

   a. _____

   b. _____

   c. _____

WORKBOOK EXERCISES

Chapter 16 Introduction to Dental Imaging Examinations

MATCHING

Basic Terminology

A. bite-wing receptor

B. dentulous

C. edentulous

D. extraoral receptor

E. intraoral receptor

F. mandible

G. maxilla

H. occlude

I. occlusal receptor

J. occlusion

K. periapical receptor

L. panoramic

_E_ 1. receptor placed inside of the mouth

_D_ 2. receptor placed outside of the mouth

_I_ 3. receptor used to examine a large area of the maxilla or mandible

_A_ 4. receptor used to examine the crowns of the upper and lower teeth

_K_ 5. receptor used to examine the entire tooth and supporting bone

_F_ 6. lower jaw

_G_ 7. upper jaw

_H_ 8. to close or to bite

_B_ 9. with teeth

_C_ 10. without teeth

_L_ 11. image used to examine large areas of the maxilla and mandible, as well as adjacent structures

Kelsey Rubin

Prescribing of Dental Images

1. Review Table 5-1 in Chapter 5 of your textbook. For each example below, list the dental images that are needed based on the ADA guidelines.

   a. Adult—new patient: individualized radiographic exame consisting of posterior bite wings w/ panoramic exam or posterior bite-wings + selected periapical images

   b. Adult—recall patient with no caries risk: Posterior bite-wing exam at 24-to 36-month intervals

   c. Adult—recall patient at risk for caries: Posterior bite-wing exam at 6-to 18-month intervals

   d. Adult—recall patient with periodontal disease: Clinical judgement needed based on eval of perio disease, maybe bitwing periapical image.

2. List the five criteria for a diagnostic intraoral image.

   a. Paralleling

   b. bisecting

   c. bite-wing

   d. Occlusal

   e. respectively

WORKBOOK EXERCISES

Chapter 17   Paralleling Technique

BASIC TERMINOLOGY CROSSWORD PUZZLE

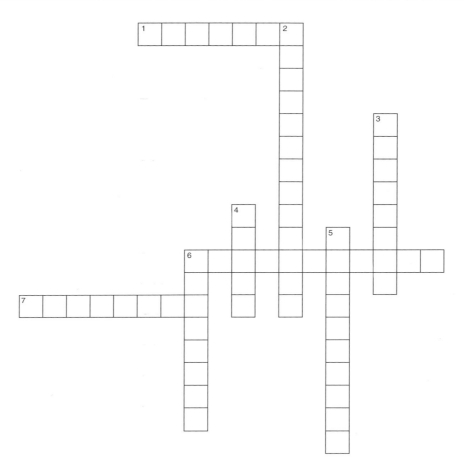

ACROSS

1   a type of beam alignment device that is used with the paralleling technique; these include plastic bite blocks, plastic aiming rings, and metal indicator arms

6   an intraoral imaging technique used to expose periapical receptors; the receptor is placed parallel to the long axis of the tooth; the central ray is directed perpendicular to the receptor and the long axis of tooth; a beam alignment device must be used to keep the receptor parallel to the long axis of the tooth

7   something that responds to a stimulus; a recording medium; examples: x-ray film or digital sensors

DOWN

2   intersecting at or forming right angles

3   an imaginary line that divides a tooth longitudinally into two equal halves

4   a bony growth in the oral cavity

5   central portion of the primary beam of x-radiation

6   moving or lying in the same plane; always separated by the same distance and not intersecting

DRAWING EXERCISE

Basic Concepts

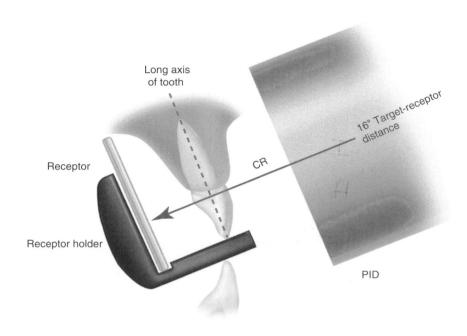

Indicate the 90-degree angle formed by each of the following by drawing a ■ on the diagram above.

1. biting surface of bite block   — and —   long axis of tooth
2. biting surface of bite block   — and —   receptor
3. CR   — and —   receptor
4. CR   — and —   long axis of tooth
5. CR   — and —   opening of PID

MULTIPLE CHOICE

Parallel vs. Perpendicular

Circle the correct answer.

1. receptor is   **parallel / perpendicular**   to the CR
2. receptor is   **parallel / perpendicular**   to the long axis of tooth
3. receptor is   **parallel / perpendicular**   to the biting surface of bite block
4. receptor is   **parallel / perpendicular**   to the opening of the PID
5. CR is   **parallel / perpendicular**   to the receptor
6. CR is   **parallel / perpendicular**   to the long axis of tooth
7. CR is   **parallel / perpendicular**   to the biting surface of bite block
8. CR is   **parallel / perpendicular**   to the opening of the PID

RINN Devices

Circle the correct answers for Fig. 17-1.

1. **anterior** RINN   **posterior** RINN
2. **size 1** receptor   **size 2** receptor
3. receptor placed **vertically**   receptor placed **horizontally**
4. if using film, **dot in slot**   if using film, **dot opposite slot**

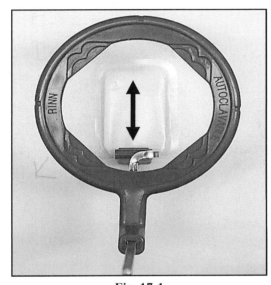

Fig. 17-1

Circle the correct answers for Fig. 17-2.

5. **anterior** RINN   **posterior** RINN
6. **size 1** receptor   **size 2** receptor
7. receptor placed **vertically**   receptor placed **horizontally**
8. if using film, **dot** in slot   if using film, **dot opposite slot**

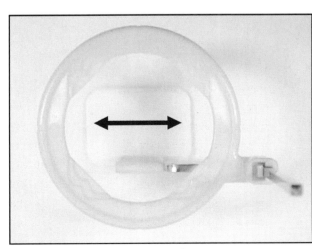

Fig. 17-2

   Module **3** **Radiographer and Technique Basics**

Periapical Receptor Placement — Anterior Exposure Sequence

Draw each **ANTERIOR** periapical receptor placement and label with the **exposure sequence numbers** (1-7) listed below.

Starting on the patient's right, draw an outline of a size 1 receptor centered on the max R canine to represent the first exposure, exposure 1. Next, note the outline around the max R lateral-central. This is the second exposure and is labeled as exposure 2. Continue drawing each anterior receptor placement with its corresponding exposure sequence number.

Refer to Table 17-1 on page 156 of text.

1. max R   canine
2. max R   lat-central
3. max L   central-lat
4. max L   canine
5. man L   canine
6. man   incisors
7. man R   canine

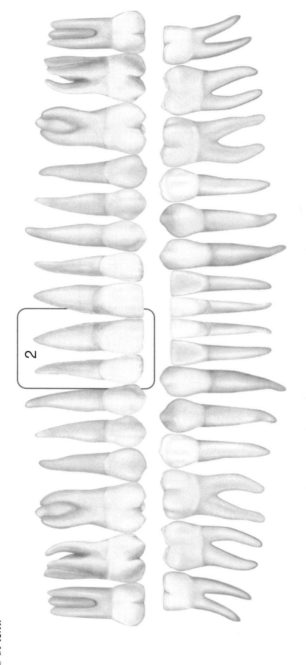

Module 3   **Radiographer and Technique Basics**

Periapical Receptor Placement – Posterior Exposure Sequence

Draw each POSTERIOR periapical receptor placement and label with the **exposure sequence numbers** (1-8) listed below. Start on the patient's right and end on the patient's right. For all posterior exposures, expose the premolars in each quadrant before the molars.

Draw an outline of a size 2 receptor around the max R premolars to represent the first exposure, exposure 1. Continue drawing each posterior receptor placement with its corresponding exposure sequence number. Note the last exposure, the mand R molar, is drawn and labeled as exposure 8. Refer to Table 17-2 on page 159 of text.

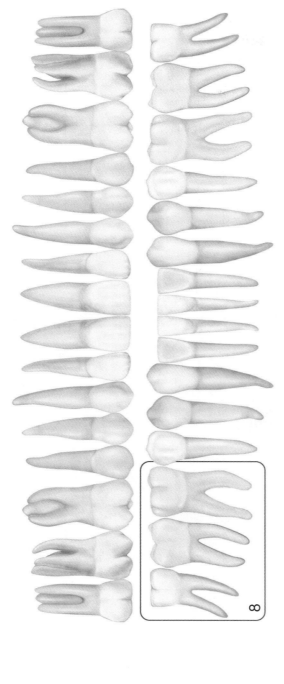

1. max R   premolar
2. max R   molar
3. man L   premolar
4. man L   molar
5. max L   premolar
6. max L   molar
7. man R   premolar
8. man R   molar

Module **3** **Radiographer and Technique Basics**

Evaluate each image. Mark each item that is visible with a check mark (✔).

MAXILLARY PERIAPICALS

Molar	Premolar	Canine	Incisor
___ front edge is in middle of 2nd premolar	___ front edge is in middle of canine	___ canine centered	___ lateral and central centered
___ all molars visible	___ all premolars visible	___ canine visible	___ lateral and central visible
___ 2–3 mm around apices	___ 2–3 mm around apices	___ 2–3 mm around apex	___ 2–3 mm around apices
___ airspace along crowns	___ airspace along crowns	___ airspace along crowns	___ airspace along crowns
___ open contacts	___ open contacts	___ open contact between canine and lateral only	___ open contacts
___ occlusal plane parallel	___ occlusal plane parallel		

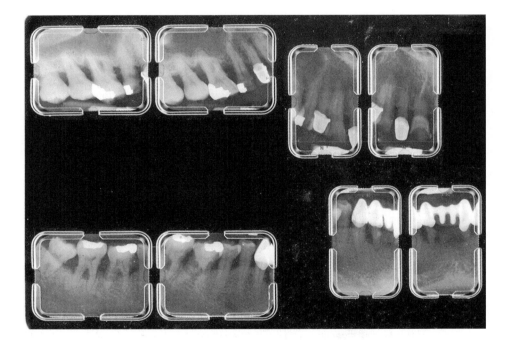

MANDIBULAR PERIAPICALS

Molar	Premolar	Canine	Incisor
___ front edge is in middle of 2nd premolar	___ front edge is in middle of canine	___ canine centered	___ midline centered
___ all molars visible	___ all premolars visible	___ canine visible	___ all incisors visible
___ 2–3 mm around apices	___ 2–3 mm around apices	___ 2–3 mm around apex	___ 2–3 mm around apices
___ airspace along crowns	___ airspace along crowns	___ airspace along crowns	___ airspace along crowns
___ open contacts	___ open contacts	___ open contact between canine and lateral only	___ open contacts
___ occlusal plane parallel	___ occlusal plane parallel		

Evaluate each image. Mark each item that is visible with a check mark (✔).

MAXILLARY PERIAPICALS

Molar	Premolar	Canine	Incisor
___ front edge is in middle of 2nd premolar	___ front edge is in middle of canine	___ canine centered	___ lateral and central centered
___ all molars visible	___ all premolars visible	___ canine visible	___ lateral and central visible
___ 2–3 mm around apices	___ 2–3 mm around apices	___ 2–3 mm around apex	___ 2–3 mm around apices
___ airspace along crowns	___ airspace along crowns	___ airspace along crowns	___ airspace along crowns
___ open contacts	___ open contacts	___ open contact between canine and lateral only	___ open contacts
___ occlusal plane parallel	___ occlusal plane parallel		

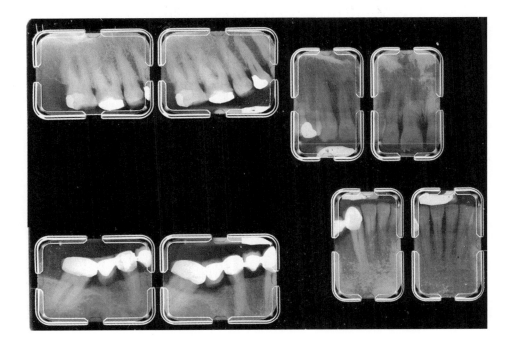

MANDIBULAR PERIAPICALS

Molar	Premolar	Canine	Incisor
___ front edge is in middle of 2nd premolar	___ front edge is in middle of canine	___ canine centered	___ midline centered
___ all molars visible	___ all premolars visible	___ canine visible	___ all incisors visible
___ 2–3 mm around apices	___ 2–3 mm around apices	___ 2–3 mm around apex	___ 2–3 mm around apices
___ airspace along crowns	___ airspace along crowns	___ airspace along crowns	___ airspace along crowns
___ open contacts	___ open contacts	___ open contact between canine and lateral only	___ open contacts
___ occlusal plane parallel	___ occlusal plane parallel		

Evaluate each image. Mark each item that is visible with a check mark (✔).

MAXILLARY PERIAPICALS

Molar	Premolar	Canine	Incisor
___ front edge is in middle of 2nd premolar	___ front edge is in middle of canine	___ canine centered	___ lateral and central centered
___ all molars visible	___ all premolars visible	___ canine visible	___ lateral and central visible
___ 2–3 mm around apices	___ 2–3 mm around apices	___ 2–3 mm around apex	___ 2–3 mm around apices
___ airspace along crowns	___ airspace along crowns	___ airspace along crowns	___ airspace along crowns
___ open contacts	___ open contacts	___ open contact between canine and lateral only	___ open contacts
___ occlusal plane parallel	___ occlusal plane parallel		

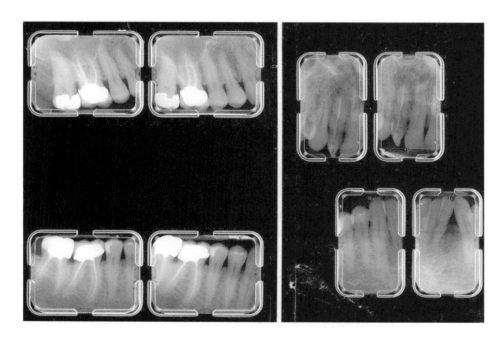

MANDIBULAR PERIAPICALS

Molar	Premolar	Canine	Incisor
___ front edge is in middle of 2nd premolar	___ front edge is in middle of canine	___ canine centered	___ midline centered
___ all molars visible	___ all premolars visible	___ canine visible	___ all incisors visible
___ 2–3 mm around apices	___ 2–3 mm around apices	___ 2–3 mm around apex	___ 2–3 mm around apices
___ airspace along crowns	___ airspace along crowns	___ airspace along crowns	___ airspace along crowns
___ open contacts	___ open contacts	___ open contact between canine and lateral only	___ open contacts
___ occlusal plane parallel	___ occlusal plane parallel		

APPLICATION

Module 3 Radiographer and Technique Basics

SELF-ASSESSMENT

Chapters 11 – 17

Based on the worksheets that you have just completed for Chapters 11 - 17, how prepared are you for the upcoming Module 3 assessments?

_____ very prepared, confident

_____ somewhat prepared, somewhat confident

_____ somewhat unprepared, lack confidence

_____ unprepared, no confidence

Based on your answer above, what is your plan for improvement? List the topics and concepts that you need to further review and study for assessments.

_____

_____

_____

_____

_____

_____

CRITICAL THINKING QUESTIONS

What does all the information in Chapters 11 to 17 mean to you in the practice setting? Use the questions below to help yu apply the information that you have just learned. Work in pairs and practice answering these questions with your classmates. Share feedback concerning the content and delivery of information—is the information correct and understandable for the average patient? Are effective communication skills being used? The more you practice, the more comfortable you will be discussing these issues with your patients.

1. **A new patient tells you, "This sure does seem like a lot of x-rays to have taken in one visit." How would you respond to the patient?**

   • CHAPTER 11

2. **Your employer asks you what you plan to do to improve your imaging skills. Discuss your goals for becoming a competent radiographer.**

   • CHAPTER 11

3. **You are about to meet a new patient for the first time. What do you plan to say as a first greeting?**

   • CHAPTER 12

4. **A patient has been a regular in your dental office for 3 years, getting examinations and cleanings every year. The patient calls your office and states he has a toothache. You inform the patient that he must come to the office for an evaluation by the dentist. When the patient arrives you notice there are entries made in the progress notes that this patient will not allow dental images to be taken. How would you handle this situation?**

   • CHAPTER 13

5. **A new patient comes into your office for a checkup. He has come to your office because he was very unhappy that the previous dentist would not give him a copy of his dental images. The previous dentist said that the patient had no rights to the images. The patient is very upset and feels misled. What can you do to help this patient?**

   • CHAPTER 14

6. **A new patient observes you placing plastic barriers. The patient tells you, "Isn't this overkill? I don't have any diseases." How would you respond to this patient about infection control?**

   • CHAPTER 15

7. **You are about to take a complete mouth series on a new patient. The patient asks you "How is the decision made to take all of these x-rays? Does every patient have this done?" How would you respond to this patient?**

   • CHAPTER 16

8. **A patient comes into the clinic needing a full series of images. You will use the paralleling technique on her, but she has a large palatal torus. How will you modify your technique to accommodate this torus?**

   • CHAPTER 17

TO-DO CHECKLIST

Written Exercises

_____ Complete all worksheets.

_____ Complete periapical assessment exercises.

_____ Complete self-assessment.

Active Learning Experiences

_____ Assemble both RINN devices.

_____ Demonstrate proper placement of receptor in both RINN devices.

_____ Using a typodont, demonstrate receptor placement using the paralleling technique.

_____ Practice answering critical thinking questions with your classmates and provide feedback.

Clinical Laboratory Activities

_____ Complete activities in Section 2, _Laboratory Manual (as assigned by instructor)._

Assessments

_____ Complete assessments in Section 2, _Laboratory Manual (as assigned by instructor)._

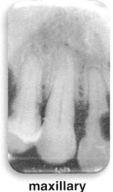
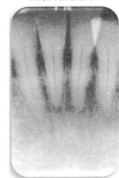

mandibular **maxillary**

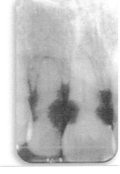

PARALLELING TECHNIQUE REVIEW

PERIAPICAL CHECKLIST

Canine

____ canine positioned in center of receptor

____ 2 to 3 mm beyond apex visible

____ maxillary—will see overlap of 1st premolar

____ no cone-cuts

____ no exposure, handling, or processing errors

Incisor

____ maxillary—center on central/lateral contact area

____ mandibular—center on midline

____ 2 to 3 mm beyond apex visible

____ no cone-cuts

____ no exposure, handling, or processing errors

Molar

____ front edge in middle of 2nd premolar

____ molars visible

____ 2 to 3 mm beyond molar apices visible

____ occlusal plane parallel with film edge

____ correct horizontal = open molar contacts

____ no cone-cuts

____ no exposure, handling, or processing errors

Premolar

____ front edge in middle of canine

____ premolars visible

____ 2 to 3 mm beyond premolar apices visible

____ occlusal plane parallel with film edge

____ correct horizontal = open premolar contacts

____ no cone-cuts

____ no exposure, handling, or processing errors

maxillary

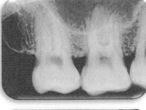
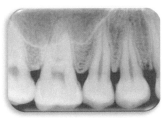

mandibular

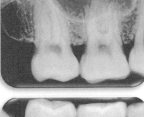
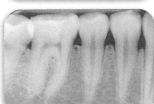
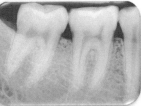

TEACHING MANIKIN OVERVIEW

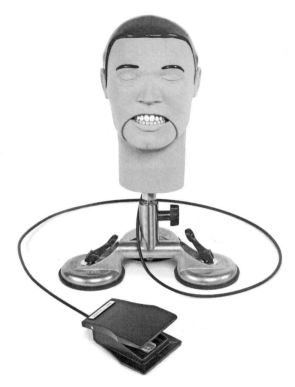

In your clinical experiences, you will expose and produce dental images utilizing a teaching manikin known as **DXTTR** (dental x-ray training and teaching replica).

DXTTR (pronounced "dexter") is a dental x-ray training and teaching manikin developed under the sponsorship of the Bureau of Radiologic Health of the Food and Drug Administration for the purpose of teaching and demonstrating proper radiographic positioning. DXTTR is the most realistic patient manikin available for use in intraoral dental imaging.

The DXTTR manikin:

- includes life like open and closing movements of the mouth;

- is ideal for positioning and exposure of intraoral receptors;

- allows for unlimited imaging exposures;

- eliminates patient variables, making it easier to evaluate student technique results; and

- allows for comparisons of various placements and projections.

Some DXTTR units are "hands free" and controlled with foot pedals, whereas others require the use of a lever-and-ratchet mechanism to open and close the mouth. Some DXTTR units are designed to be used in a dental chair, whereas others are used with a table top stand.

Each DXTTR is very expensive and must be used with care to avoid damage and costly repairs. Before use, instructors are advised to demonstrate how DXTTR functions.

116

NUMBERS REVIEW

CHAPTERS 11 TO 23

3 types	**intraoral examinations** (periapical, bite-wing, occlusal)
5 to 15 degrees	amount to **increase vertical angulation** if shallow palate
2 to 3 mm	on a periapical image, minimum amount **beyond apex**
1/8 inch	amount of film beyond incisal edge in **bisecting** technique
14 to 20	number of films in a **complete series**
15-16	number of PAs exposed with **paralleling** technique
14	number of PAs needed for an **edentulous patient**
14	number of PAs exposed with **bisecting technique**
7-8	number of **anterior** PAs used in **paralleling** technique
6	number of **anterior** PAs used in **bisecting** technique
8	number of **posterior** PAs used in **paralleling** technique
8	number of **posterior** PAs used in **bisecting** technique
7	number of **vertical BWs** (3 anterior + 4 posterior)
sizes 0, 2, 3	receptor size choices for **BW examination**
sizes 2, 4	receptor size choices for **occlusal examination**
+10 degrees	**vertical angulation - all BWs** (horizontal and vertical)
+60 degrees	**vertical angulation - maxillary pediatric** occlusal
−55 degrees	**vertical angulation - mandibular pediatric** occlusal
90 degrees	**vertical angulation - mandibular cross sectional** occlusal

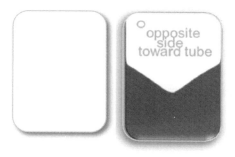

FILM

- **white side** (tube side) faces the PID
- **WHITE** in **SIGHT**

ANTERIOR RINN DEVICE
maxillary and **mandibular**

- **size 1 receptor** is placed **vertically**
- **anterior RINN** is assembled like this for <u>both</u> maxillary and mandibular placements
- <u>no</u> reassembly is needed

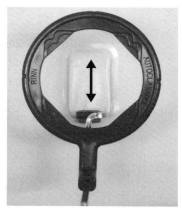

POSTERIOR RINN DEVICE
maxillary right and mandibular left

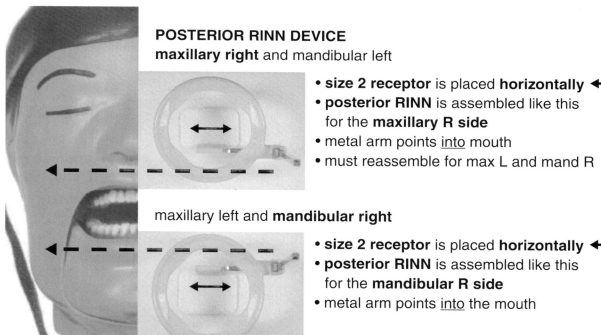

- **size 2 receptor** is placed **horizontally**
- **posterior RINN** is assembled like this for the **maxillary R side**
- metal arm points <u>into</u> mouth
- must reassemble for max L and mand R

maxillary left and **mandibular right**

- **size 2 receptor** is placed **horizontally**
- **posterior RINN** is assembled like this for the **mandibular R side**
- metal arm points <u>into</u> the mouth

INSTRUCTIONS

How to Prepare
- Review the learning objectives for Module 4 prior to lab.
- Review the critical thinking questions for Module 4 prior to lab.

What to Bring
- *Workbook and Laboratory Manual*—Module 4 materials
- pencil
- textbook (print or e-version)
- typodont

Written Exercises
- Work together or individually to complete each exercise.
- For each chapter, complete the worksheets in pencil (*without looking up answers*).
- When each exercise is finished, use your text to check answers; correct any wrong answers.
- Use your completed and corrected packet to study for assessments.

Active Learning Experiences
- Practice assembly of bite-wing RINN device.
- Practice receptor placements utilizing the bite-wing technique on a typodont.
- In pairs, take turns answering each critical thinking question and provide feedback to each other.
- Ask your instructor to observe you answering the critical thinking questions and provide you with feedback.

Clinical Laboratory Activities
- See Section 2, *Laboratory Manual.*

Assessments
- See Section 2, *Laboratory Manual.*

Technique Basics

LEARNING OBJECTIVES

The goal of Module 4 laboratory experiences is to provide students with a reinforcement of the fundamental understanding of technique basics. Upon successful completion of Chapters 18 to 24 lectures and laboratory, the student will be able to:

CHAPTER	LEARNING OBJECTIVES
CHAPTER 18 BISECTING TECHNIQUE	
Written Exercises	• Summarize the principles of the bisecting technique. • Describe how elongated and foreshortened images occur and how to correct these errors.
CHAPTER 19 BITE-WING TECHNIQUE	
Written Exercises	• Describe the basic concepts and purpose of the bite-wing image. • Describe the horizontal/vertical angulations and procedures for horizontal bite-wings. • Discuss the purpose and use of vertical bite-wing images. • Recognize common bite-wing errors and discuss how to correct each error.
Active Learning Experiences	• Assemble the bite-wing RINN, demonstrate receptor placement in the RINN, demonstrate placement of receptor and RINN using typodont, place tab on bite-wing receptor.
CHAPTER 20 EXPOSURE AND TECHNIQUE ERRORS	
Written Exercises	• Describe and identify exposure and technique errors. • Discuss solutions for exposure and technique errors.
CHAPTER 21 OCCLUSAL AND LOCALIZATION TECHNIQUES	
Written Exercises	• Define basic terminology used with the occlusal technique and buccal object rule. • Describe the basic concepts and step-by-step procedures for occlusal and buccal object rule. • Recognize vertical angulations for common occlusal projections. • Using the buccal object rule, identify item as buccal or lingual. • Describe what SLOB refers to with the buccal object rule.
CHAPTER 22 PANORAMIC IMAGING	
Written Exercises (more exercises in Module 6)	• Review panoramic patient preparation and positioning checklist. • Recognize common panoramic errors and discuss how to correct each error.

CHAPTER	LEARNING OBJECTIVES

CHAPTER 23   EXTRAORAL IMAGING

Written Exercises

- Define basic terminology used with extraoral imaging.
- Identify the specific purposes of each extraoral imaging technique.
- Describe the purpose of a grid used in extraoral imaging.

CHAPTER 24   IMAGING OF PATIENTS WITH SPECIAL NEEDS

Written Exercises

- Summarize problems encountered in dealing with patients with special needs.
- Describe how to manage the imaging needs of patients with a hypersensitive gag reflex, patients with physical or developmental disabilities, endodontic patients, and edentulous patients.
- Identify the eruption timeline for all permanent teeth.
- Identify what permanent tooth replaces each primary tooth.
- Label each primary tooth A – T.
- Identify the approximate age of a patient based on what teeth are present.

MODULE 4   CLINICAL LABORATORY ACTIVITIES

- Apply information learned to complete activities in Section 2, *Laboratory Manual* (as assigned by instructor).

MODULE 4   ASSESSMENTS

- Apply information learned to complete assessments in Section 2, *Laboratory Manual* (as assigned by instructor).

WORKBOOK EXERCISES

Chapter 18   Bisecting Technique

IDENTIFY AND DESCRIBE

Bisecting Technique

1. Identify each item labeled in Fig. 18-1.

    A. _____

    B. _____

    C. _____

    D. _____

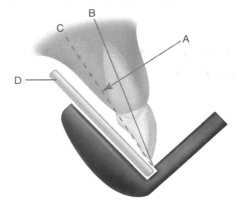

Fig. 18-1

2. State the principles of the bisecting technique. _____

_____

_____

_____

_____

PID Angulation

1. Identify the angulation error in Fig. 18-2. _____

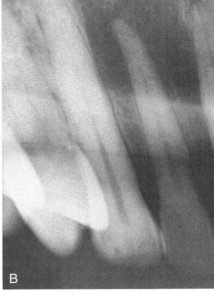

Fig. 18-2

123

2. Identify the angulation error in Fig. 18-3. _____

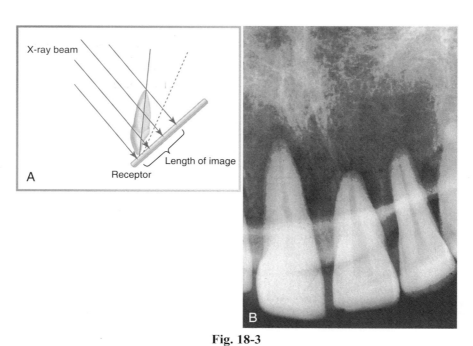

Fig. 18-3

MULTIPLE CHOICE

Elongation and Foreshortening

Circle the correct answer.

1. **ELONGATION**   is caused by using   **too much / too little**   vertical angulation
2. **FORESHORTENING** is caused by using   **too much / too little**   vertical angulation
3. **ELONGATION**   is caused by using   **too steep / too flat**   vertical angulation
4. **FORESHORTENING** is caused by using   **too steep / too flat**   vertical angulation
5. **ELONGATION**   can be corrected by   **increasing / decreasing**   vertical angulation
6. **FORESHORTENING** can be corrected by   **increasing / decreasing**   vertical angulation
7. **Vertical / Horizontal** angulation is the positioning of the PID in an up-and-down plane
8. **Vertical / Horizontal** angulation is the positioning of the PID in a side-to-side plane
9. **Vertical / Horizontal** angulation does not differ according to the technique used

Name _Kelsey Rubin_
Date _10-12-20_

WORKBOOK EXERCISES

Chapter 19   Bite-Wing Technique

COMPLETION

Basic Concepts

1. The bite-wing technique is used to examine the _interproximal_ surfaces of teeth.

2. Bite-wing images are also used to examine the level of _crestal_ bone.

3. Describe the basic principles of the bite-wing technique (use Fig. 19-1 as a guide).

   1. receptor is placed in the mouth parrell to the completely crowns of both max + man 2. stablized 3. verticial angulation of 10+ degrees

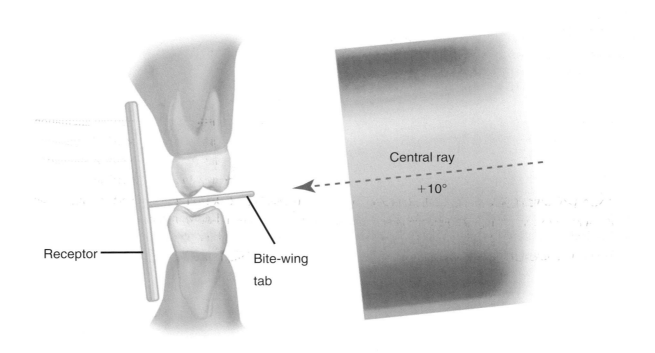

Receptor ——

Central ray

+10°

Bite-wing
tab

Fig. 19-1

Kelsey Rubin

Horizontal Angulation

1. Using the diagram in Fig. 19-2, draw the PID (edge of cone) for the PREMOLAR bite-wing.

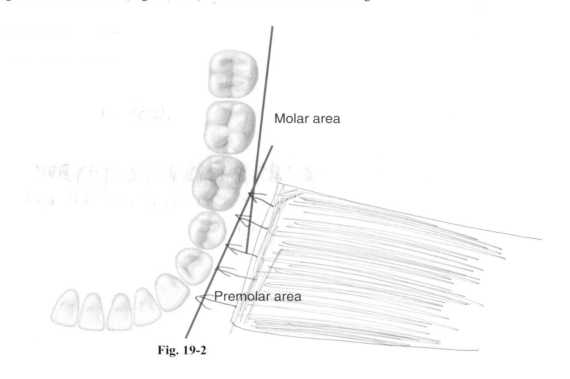

Molar area

Premolar area

Fig. 19-2

2. Using the diagram in Fig. 19-3, draw the PID (edge of cone) for the MOLAR bite-wing.
   *See Figs. 19-22 and 19-16 in your textbook for examples.

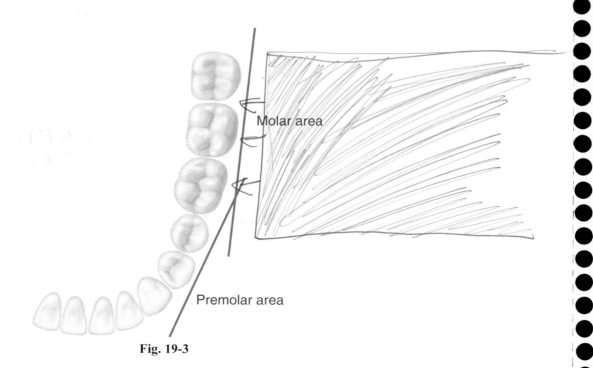

Molar area

Premolar area

Fig. 19-3

Receptor Placement

1. On Fig. 19-4, draw the ideal receptor placement for the PREMOLAR bite-wing.

2. Where should the front edge of the receptor be positioned? <u>at the canine middle of lower mandibular</u>

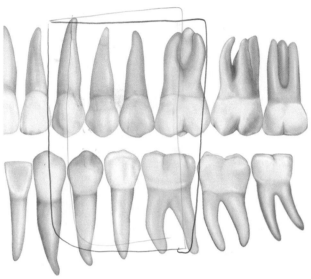

Fig. 19-4

3. On Fig. 19-5, draw the ideal receptor placement for the MOLAR bite-wing.

4. Where should the front edge of the receptor be positioned? <u>at the middle of lower mandibular 2nd premolar</u>

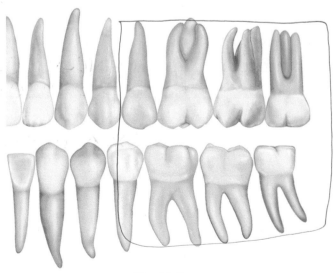

Fig. 19-5

MULTIPLE CHOICE AND SHORT ANSWER

Vertical Angulation

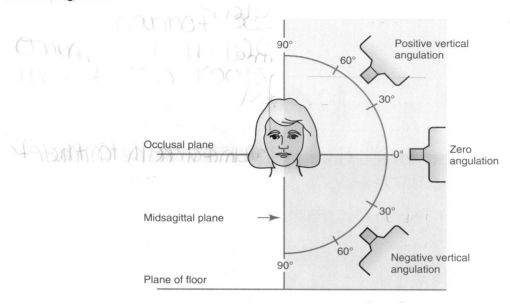

Circle the correct answer.

1. posterior bite-wings require   **positive** / **negative**   vertical angulation

2. anterior bite-wings require   **positive** / **negative**   vertical angulation

3. the PID is directed   **up** / **down**   for anterior bite-wings

4. the PID is directed   **up** / **down**   for posterior bite-wings

5. vertical angulation is   **+10 degrees** / **–10 degrees**   for all bite-wings

Bite-Wing Exposure Sequence

Circle the correct answer.

1. On each side of the arch, the bite-wing exposure sequence is **premolar then molar** / **molar then premolar.**

2. List the rationale for the bite-wing exposure sequence.

1. expose all anterior periapical receptors
2. follow w/ exposure of posterior periapical receptors
3. finish w/ bite wing exposures.

Kelsey Rubin
10-12-20

IDENTIFICATION AND SHORT ANSWER

Bite-Wing Errors

1. Identify the error on the bite-wing in Fig. 19-6.

   none?

2. Identify how to correct the error in Fig. 19-6.

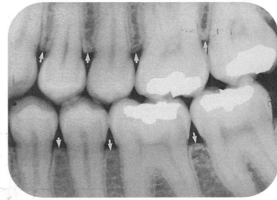

Fig. 19-6

3. Identify the error on the bite-wing in Fig. 19-7.

   incorrect Horizontal Angulation

4. Identify how to correct the error in Fig. 19-7.

   -overlapping -interproximal spaces unclear

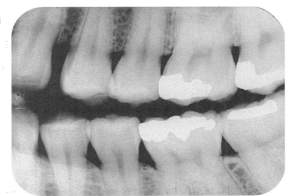

Fig. 19-7

5. Is the bite-wing in Fig. 19-8 placed properly?

   no

6. Why or why not?

   does not include the third molar through the distal portion of the second premolar

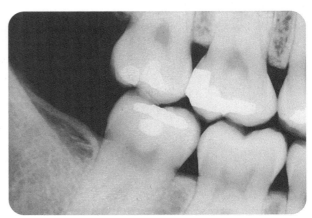

Fig. 19-8

Module **4** **Technique Basics**

Name Kelsey Rubin

Date _____

7. Is the bite-wing in Fig. 19-9 placed properly?

_____ yes _____

8. Why or why not? cannot see
enough of both the
max + man roots

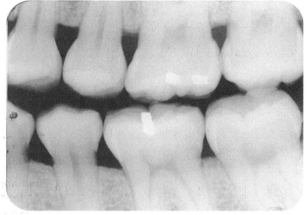

Fig. 19-9

Module **4** Technique Basics

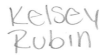
Kelsey
Rubin

INSTRUCTIONS FOR BITE-WING TECHNIQUE ASSESSMENT EXERCISES

- Evaluate each bite-wing image using the criteria listed.

- You may use the criteria listed with bite-wing images provided in your laboratory.

- Mark each item that is correct with a check mark (✔).

- Practice writing a patient record entry concerning each set of bite-wings (see example below).

Date	ADA Procedure Code	Provider	Charting Notes	Comments
3/13/16	0274	LJH	Dr. Campbell prescribed four horizontal bite-wing exposures; digital CCD sensors used (four total exposures)	Patient recently had orthodontic appliances removed; slight cone-cut on the left premolar bite-wing, but information is present on the left molar projection.

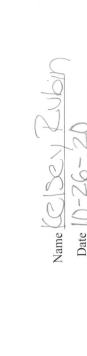

Name *Kelsey Rubin*

Date *10-26-20*

BITE-WING TECHNIQUE ASSESSMENT EXERCISE 1

BITE-WING IMAGES

Molar (right)	**Premolar (right)**
___ front edge in middle of lower 2nd premolar	___ front edge in middle of lower canine
✓ ALL molars visible	✓ ALL premolars visible
___ third molar area visible	
✓ vertical angulation +10	✓ vertical angulation +10
✓ horizontal = open contacts	✓ horizontal = open contacts
✓ occlusal plane centered and parallel with edge	✓ occlusal plane centered and parallel with edge
✓ no cone-cut	✓ no cone-cut

Premolar (left)	**Molar (left)**
✓ front edge in middle of lower canine	___ front edge in middle of lower 2nd premolar
✓ ALL premolars visible	✓ ALL molars visible
	___ third molar area visible
✓ vertical angulation +10	✓ vertical angulation +10
✓ horizontal = open contacts	✓ horizontal = open contacts
✓ occlusal plane centered and parallel with edge	✓ occlusal plane centered and parallel with edge
✓ no cone-cut	✓ no cone-cut

L

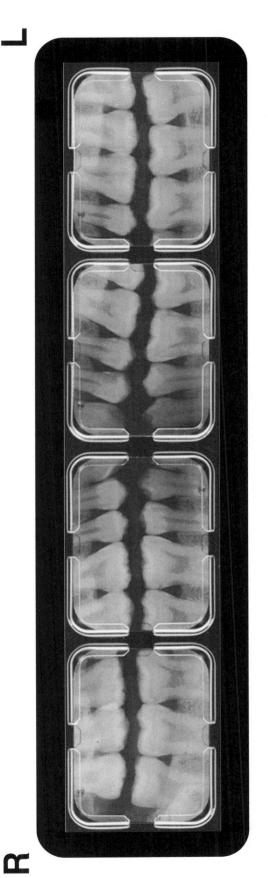

R

Kelsey Rubin

BITE-WING TECHNIQUE ASSESSMENT EXERCISE 2

BITE-WING IMAGES

Molar (right)	Premolar (right)	Premolar (left)	Molar (left)
front edge in middle of lower 2nd premolar	front edge in middle of lower canine	front edge in middle of lower canine	front edge in middle of lower 2nd premolar
ALL molars visible	ALL premolars visible	ALL premolars visible	ALL molars visible
third molar area visible			third molar area visible
vertical angulation +10	vertical angulation +10	vertical angulation +10	vertical angulation +10
horizontal = open contacts	horizontal = open contacts	horizontal = open contacts	horizontal = open contacts
occlusal plane centered and parallel with edge	occlusal plane centered and parallel with edge	occlusal plane centered and parallel with edge	occlusal plane centered and parallel with edge
no cone-cut	no cone-cut	no cone-cut	no cone-cut

L

R

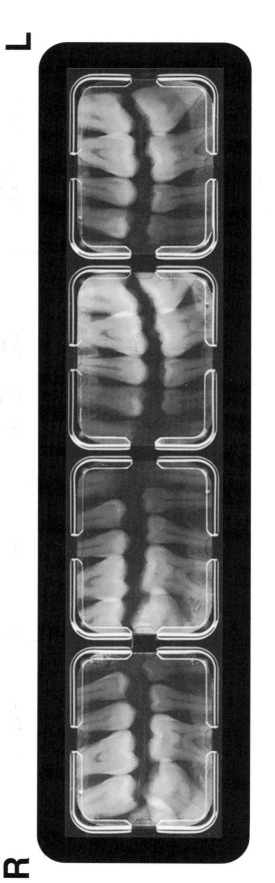

Name *Kelsey Rubin*
Date *10-26-20*

BITE-WING TECHNIQUE ASSESSMENT EXERCISE 3

BITE-WING IMAGES

Molar (right)	Premolar (right)	Premolar (left)	Molar (left)
__ front edge in middle of lower 2nd premolar	__ front edge in middle of lower canine	__ front edge in middle of lower canine	__ front edge in middle of lower 2nd premolar
__ ALL molars visible	__ ALL premolars visible	__ ALL premolars visible	__ ALL molars visible
__ third molar area visible			__ third molar area visible
__ vertical angulation +10	__ vertical angulation +10	__ vertical angulation +10	__ vertical angulation +10
__ horizontal = open contacts	__ horizontal = open contacts	__ horizontal = open contacts	__ horizontal = open contacts
__ occlusal plane centered and parallel with edge	__ occlusal plane centered and parallel with edge	__ occlusal plane centered and parallel with edge	__ occlusal plane centered and parallel with edge
__ no cone-cut	__ no cone-cut	__ no cone-cut	__ no cone-cut

L

R

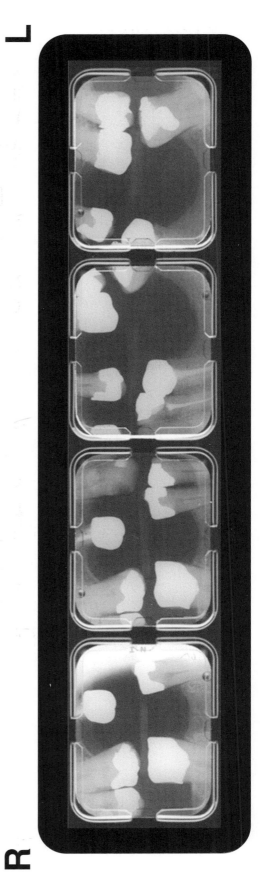

Kelsey Rubin

BITE-WING IMAGES

Molar (right)	Premolar (right)	Premolar (left)	Molar (left)
— front edge in middle of lower 2nd premolar	— front edge in middle of lower canine	— front edge in middle of lower canine	— front edge in middle of lower 2nd premolar
✓ ALL molars visible	✓ ALL premolars visible	✓ ALL premolars visible	✓ ALL molars visible
— third molar area visible			— third molar area visible
✓ vertical angulation +10	✓ vertical angulation +10	✓ vertical angulation +10	✓ vertical angulation +10
✓ horizontal = open contacts	✓ horizontal = open contacts	✓ horizontal = open contacts	✓ horizontal = open contacts
✓ occlusal plane centered and parallel with edge	✓ occlusal plane centered and parallel with edge	✓ occlusal plane centered and parallel with edge	✓ occlusal plane centered and parallel with edge
✓ no cone-cut	✓ no cone-cut	✓ no cone-cut	✓ no cone-cut

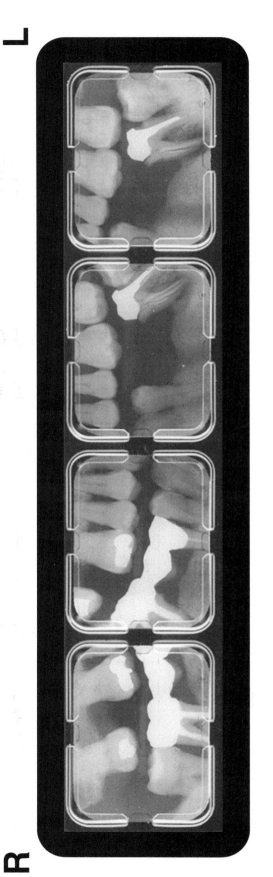

R   L

Module 4   Technique Basics

Name Kelsey Rubin
Date 10-26-20

BITE-WING TECHNIQUE ASSESSMENT EXERCISE 5

BITE-WING IMAGES

Molar (right)
- ✓ front edge in middle of lower 2nd premolar
- — ALL molars visible
- — third molar area visible
- ✓ vertical angulation +10
- ✓ horizontal = open contacts
- ✓ occlusal plane centered and parallel with edge
- ✓ no cone-cut

Premolar (right)
- — front edge in middle of lower canine
- — ALL premolars visible
- — vertical angulation +10
- ✓ horizontal = open contacts
- — occlusal plane centered and parallel with edge
- ✓ no cone-cut

Premolar (left)
- ✓ front edge in middle of lower canine
- ✓ ALL premolars visible
- — vertical angulation +10
- ✓ horizontal = open contacts
- — occlusal plane centered and parallel with edge
- ✓ no cone-cut

Molar (left)
- ✓ front edge in middle of lower 2nd premolar
- — ALL molars visible
- — third molar area visible
- ✓ vertical angulation +10
- — horizontal = open contacts
- ✓ occlusal plane centered and parallel with edge
- ✓ no cone-cut

L

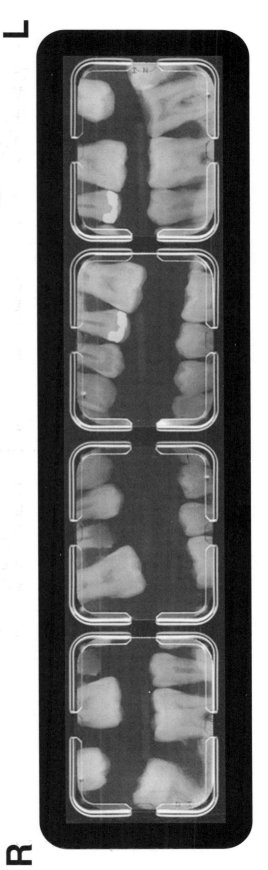

R

Kelsey Robin

BITE-WING TECHNIQUE ASSESSMENT EXERCISE 6

BITE-WING IMAGES

Molar (right)	**Premolar (right)**	**Premolar (left)**	**Molar (left)**
✓ front edge in middle of lower 2nd premolar	___ front edge in middle of lower canine	___ front edge in middle of lower canine	✓ front edge in middle of lower 2nd premolar
✓ ALL molars visible	___ ALL premolars visible	✓ ALL premolars visible	✓ ALL molars visible
___ third molar area visible			___ third molar area visible
✓ vertical angulation +10	✓ vertical angulation +10	✓ vertical angulation +10	___ vertical angulation +10
✓ horizontal = open contacts	✓ horizontal = open contacts	✓ horizontal = open contacts	___ horizontal = open contacts
✓ occlusal plane centered and parallel with edge	✓ occlusal plane centered and parallel with edge	✓ occlusal plane centered and parallel with edge	✓ occlusal plane centered and parallel with edge
✓ no cone-cut	✓ no cone-cut	✓ no cone-cut	✓ no cone-cut

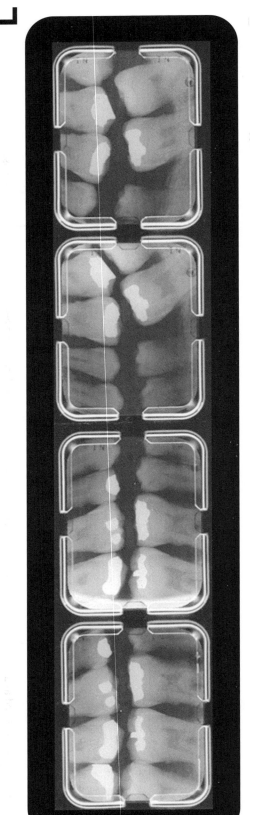

L

R

BITE-WING TECHNIQUE ASSESSMENT EXERCISE 7

Name _____

Date _____

BITE-WING IMAGES

Molar (right)	**Premolar (right)**
___ front edge in middle of lower 2nd premolar	___ front edge in middle of lower canine
___ ALL molars visible	___ ALL premolars visible
___ third molar area visible	
___ vertical angulation +10	___ vertical angulation +10
___ horizontal = open contacts	___ horizontal = open contacts
___ occlusal plane centered and parallel with edge	___ occlusal plane centered and parallel with edge
___ no cone-cut	___ no cone-cut

Premolar (left)	**Molar (left)**
___ front edge in middle of lower canine	___ front edge in middle of lower 2nd premolar
___ ALL premolars visible	___ ALL molars visible
	___ third molar area visible
___ vertical angulation +10	___ vertical angulation +10
___ horizontal = open contacts	___ horizontal = open contacts
___ occlusal plane centered and parallel with edge	___ occlusal plane centered and parallel with edge
___ no cone-cut	___ no cone-cut

R   L

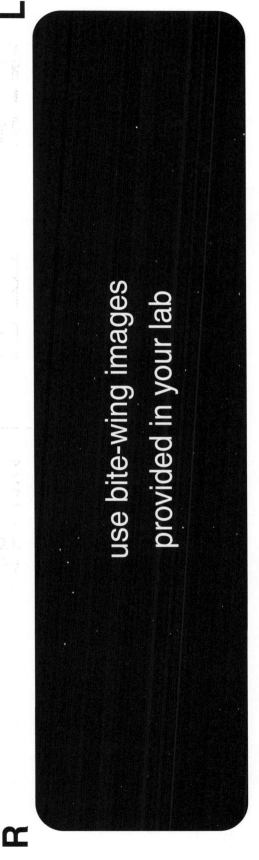

use bite-wing images
provided in your lab

BITE-WING IMAGES

Molar (right)	**Premolar (right)**	**Premolar (left)**	**Molar (left)**
___ front edge in middle of lower 2nd premolar ___ ALL molars visible ___ third molar area visible	___ front edge in middle of lower canine ___ ALL premolars visible	___ front edge in middle of lower canine ___ ALL premolars visible	___ front edge in middle of lower 2nd premolar ___ ALL molars visible ___ third molar area visible
___ vertical angulation +10 ___ horizontal = open contacts	___ vertical angulation +10 ___ horizontal = open contacts	___ vertical angulation +10 ___ horizontal = open contacts	___ vertical angulation +10 ___ horizontal = open contacts
___ occlusal plane centered and parallel with edge ___ no cone-cut	___ occlusal plane centered and parallel with edge ___ no cone-cut	___ occlusal plane centered and parallel with edge ___ no cone-cut	___ occlusal plane centered and parallel with edge ___ no cone-cut

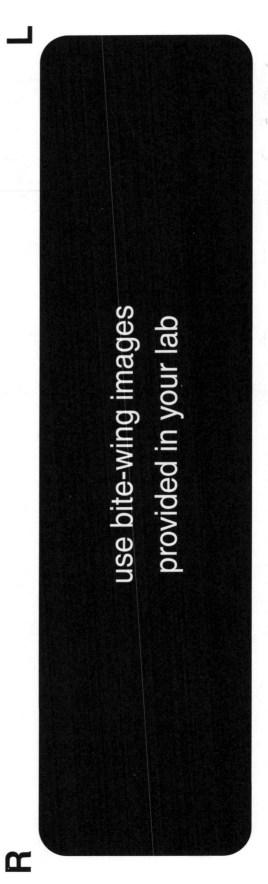

use bite-wing images
provided in your lab

R

L

WORKBOOK EXERCISES

Chapter 20   Exposure and Technique Errors

SHORT ANSWER

Explain the cause and correction for each of the exposure or technique errors in questions 1 to 12 below.

	CAUSE	CORRECTION	EXPOSURE/TECHNIQUE ERROR
1.	Underexposed	make sure KV, exposure time, is all correct	
2.	Film placed backwards	make sure film is placed correct before exposing	
3.	movement	make sure patient keeps head still, and x-ray unit arm is not moving	

Kelsey Rubin

	CAUSE	CORRECTION	EXPOSURE/TECHNIQUE ERROR
4.	incorrect placement	make sure film and receptor are inline	
5.	film crease	don't over manipulate the receptor	
6.	double exposure	film can only be exposed once	

	CAUSE	CORRECTION	EXPOSURE/TECHNIQUE ERROR
7.	vertical angulation excessive

underexposed | don't use a steep vertical angulation

make si lav. exp time ince | |
| 8. | overexposed | film was used twice and only can be exposed once | |
| 9. | insufficant vertical angulation | don't use a flat vertical angulation | |

Module **4** **Technique Basics**

Kelsey Rubin

	CAUSE	CORRECTION	EXPOSURE/TECHNIQUE ERROR
10.	incorrect placement	placement of receptor wasn't lined up with film	
11.	exposure to light	make sure film is only opened in proper dark room	
12.	Improper placement	make sure receptor is parallel to the incisalor occlusal surface of teeth	

WORKBOOK EXERCISES

Chapter 21   Occlusal and Localization Techniques

COMPLETION AND SHORT ANSWER

Occlusal Technique

1. Define occlusal.

   _____

   _____

2. What size receptor is used for an adult occlusal projection? _____

3. What size receptor is used for a pediatric occlusal projection? _____

4. How is the occlusal receptor positioned? (*principles of occlusal technique*)

   a. The tube side faces _____

   b. The receptor is placed in the mouth between the _____

   _____

   c. The receptor is stabilized when the patient _____

   _____

5. List 5 of the 10 uses for the occlusal projection:

   a. _____

   b. _____

   c. _____

   d. _____

   e. _____

6. Identify the projection in Fig. 21-1. _____

   _____

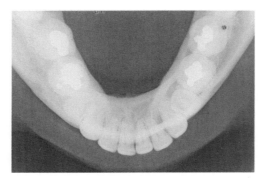

Fig. 21-1

Buccal Object Rule

1. Using the diagram in Fig. 21-2, describe the buccal object rule.

_____

_____

_____

_____

_____

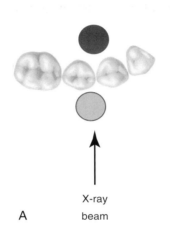

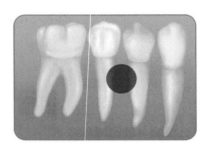

X-ray
beam

A

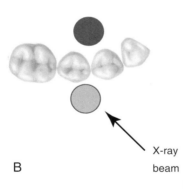

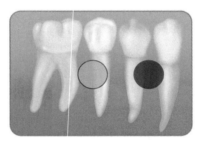

X-ray
beam

B

Fig. 21-2

MATCHING

Vertical Angulation

Some choices may be used more than once, and some choices may not be used.

A. 90 degrees   1. _____ maxillary lateral occlusal projection

B. +65 degrees   2. _____ maxillary pediatric occlusal projection

C. –65 degrees   3. _____ mandibular topographic occlusal projection

D. +55 degrees   4. _____ mandibular cross-sectional occlusal projection

E. –55 degrees   5. _____ mandibular pediatric occlusal projection

F. +60 degrees

**PA
IMAGE #1
vertical = +45**

➡

**PA
IMAGE #2
vertical = +30**

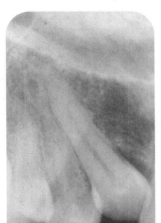

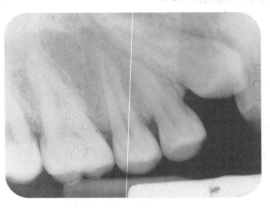

S – L – O – B
same = lingual
opposite = buccal

1. Is the canine buccal or lingual? _____

   Explain why:

   _____

   _____

   _____

2. Was the PID moved up or down? _____

3. Did the tooth move up or down? _____

BUCCAL OBJECT RULE EXERCISE 2

BW
IMAGE #1
vertical = +10

PA
IMAGE #2
vertical = −10

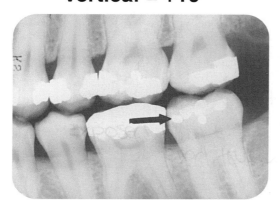 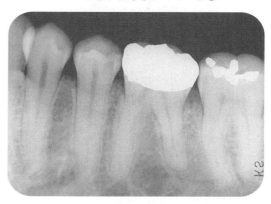

> **S – L – O – B**
> same   = lingual
> opposite = buccal

1. Is the amalgam (see arrow) buccal or lingual? _____

   Explain why:

   _____

   _____

   _____

2. Was the PID moved up or down? _____

3. Did the amalgam move up or down? _____

149

PA IMAGE #1 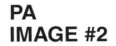 PA IMAGE #2

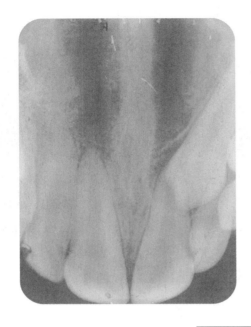
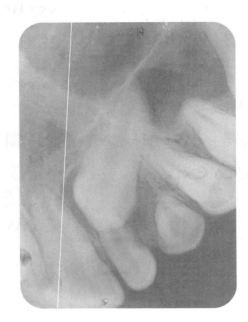

S – L – O – B

same   = lingual

opposite = buccal

1. Is the canine buccal or lingual? _____

   Explain why:

   _____

   _____

   _____

2. What direction did the PID move? _____

3. Did the tooth move in the same direction? _____

BUCCAL OBJECT RULE EXERCISE 4

**BW
IMAGE #1
vertical = +10**

**PA
IMAGE #2
vertical = −10**

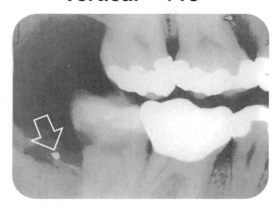 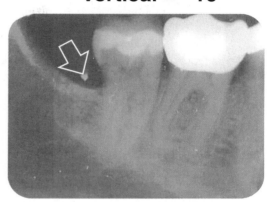

S – L – O – B
same = lingual
opposite = buccal

1. Is the amalgam (see arrow) buccal or lingual? _____

   Explain why:

   _____

   _____

   _____

2. Was the PID moved up or down? _____

3. Did the amalgam move up or down? _____

WORKBOOK EXERCISES

Chapter 22   Panoramic Imaging

IDENTIFICATION AND SHORT ANSWER

Panoramic Image #1 / Fig. 22-1

1. Identify the radiopacity (*arrow*). How can this error be avoided?

_____

_____

_____

_____

2. Identify the double images of the hyoid and the epiglottis. What causes a double image?

_____

_____

_____

_____

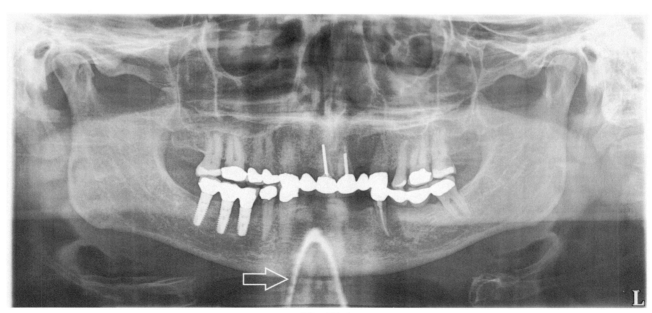

Fig. 22-1

Panoramic Image #2 / Fig. 22-2

1. Identify the head positioning error and what correction is needed.

_____

_____

_____

_____

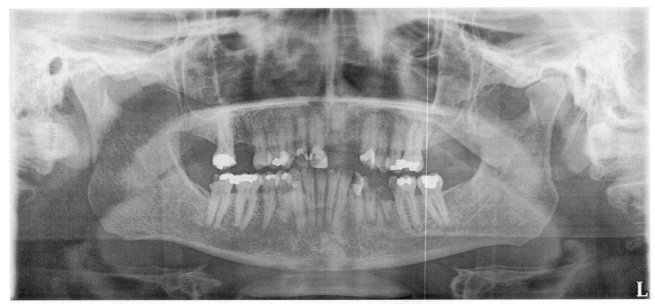

Fig. 22-2

Panoramic Image #3 / Fig. 22-3

1. Identify the head positioning error and what correction is needed.

   _____

   _____

   _____

   _____

2. Identify which side of the patient is closest to the receptor. _____

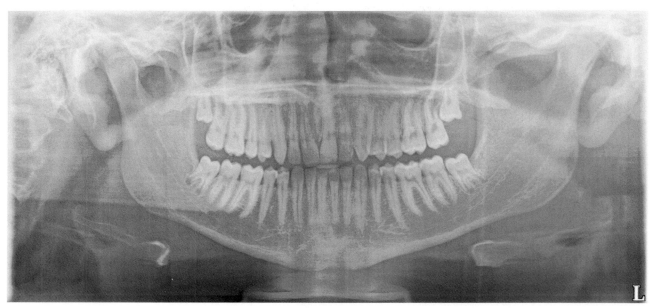

Fig. 22-3

Panoramic Image #4 / Fig. 22-4

1. Identify the head positioning error and what correction is needed.

_____

_____

_____

_____

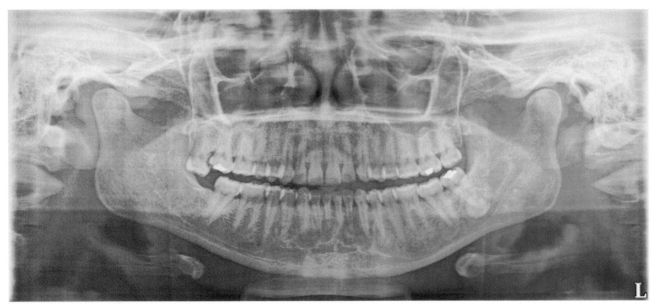

Fig. 22-4

Panoramic Image #5 / Fig. 22-5

1. Identify the tragus piercing and the related ghost image. Is this image diagnostic with this ghost image?

_____

_____

_____

_____

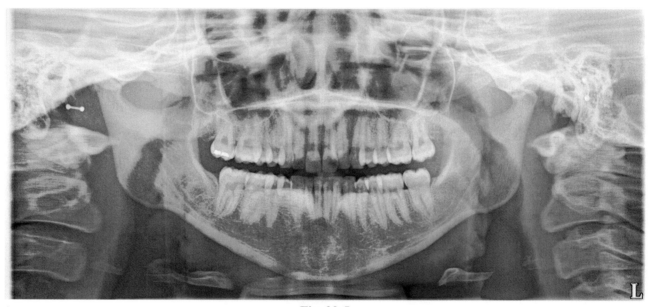

Fig. 22-5

Panoramic Image #6 / Fig. 22-6

1. Identify the head positioning error and what correction is needed.

_____

_____

_____

_____

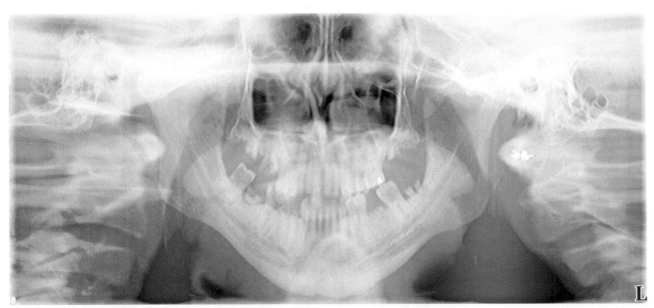

Fig. 22-6

2. Identify the focal trough error and what correction is needed.

_____

_____

_____

_____

3. Identify the ghost image of the earring on the left. Is this image diagnostic with this ghost image?

_____

_____

_____

_____

Panoramic Image #7 / Fig. 22-7

1. Identify the earrings and related ghost images. Is this image diagnostic with these ghost images?

_____

_____

_____

_____

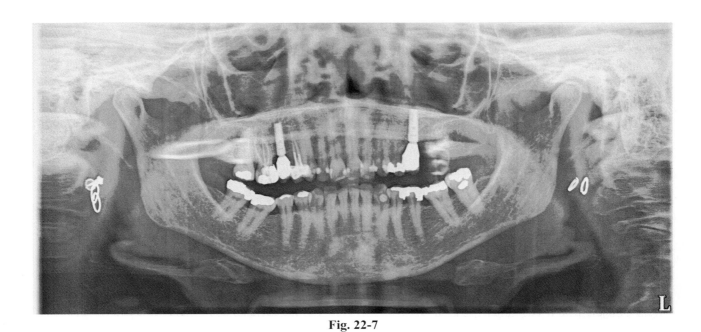

Fig. 22-7

WORKBOOK EXERCISES

Chapter 23   Extraoral Imaging

MATCHING

Extraoral Projections

A. used to evaluate maxillary sinus area

B. used to evaluate facial growth and development; often used in orthodontics

C. used to evaluate impacted teeth and fractures of body of mandible

D. used to evaluate condyle and articular eminence

E. used to identify fractures of condylar neck and ramus

F. used to evaluate trauma; demonstrates frontal sinuses, orbit, and nasal cavity

G. used to evaluate impacted teeth and fractures that extend to the ramus

H. used to identify the position of the condyles; used for zygomatic fractures

_____ 1. lateral jaw, body

_____ 2. lateral jaw, ramus

_____ 3. lateral cephalometric

_____ 4. posteroanterior

_____ 5. Waters

_____ 6. submentovertex

_____ 7. reverse Towne

_____ 8. transcranial

SHORT ANSWER

1. Define extraoral. _____

_____

2. List five uses for extraoral images.

   a. _____

   b. _____

   c. _____

   d. _____

   e. _____

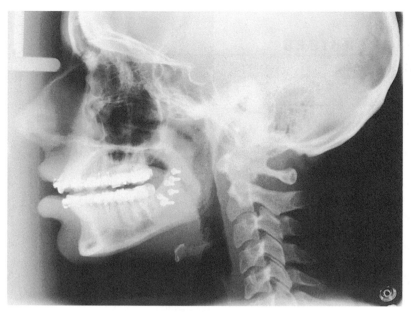

Fig. 23-1

3. Identify the projection in Fig. 23-1. _____

4. Describe the purpose of a grid (use the diagram in Fig. 23-2 as a guide).

_____

_____

_____

_____

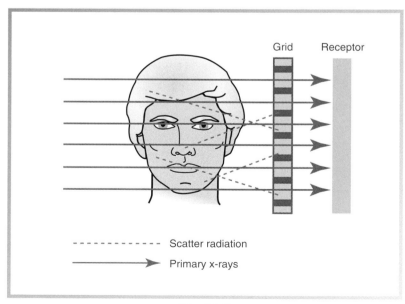

Fig. 23-2

WORKBOOK EXERCISES

Chapter 24   Imaging of Patients with Special Needs

IDENTIFICATION

Eruption of Permanent Teeth

MAXILLARY   AGE AT ERUPTION

1. incisor, central   _____

2. incisor, lateral   _____

3. canine   _____

4. premolar, first   _____

5. premolar, second   _____

6. molar, first   _____

7. molar, second   _____

8. molar, third   _____

MANDIBULAR   AGE AT ERUPTION

1. incisor, central   _____

2. incisor, lateral   _____

3. canine   _____

4. premolar, first   _____

5. premolar, second   _____

6. molar, first   _____

7. molar, second   _____

8. molar, third   _____

What permanent tooth replaces each tooth listed?

1. D   _____

2. E   _____

3. N   _____

4. T   _____

5. A   _____

6. L   _____

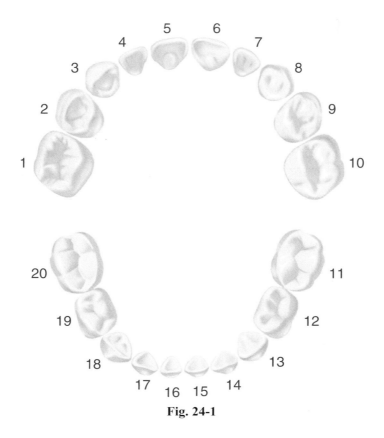

Fig. 24-1

Primary Tooth Identification

Label each primary tooth in Fig. 24-1. (using letters A through T)

1. _____   6. _____   11. _____   16. _____

2. _____   7. _____   12. _____   17. _____

3. _____   8. _____   13. _____   18. _____

4. _____   9. _____   14. _____   19. _____

5. _____   10. _____   15. _____   20. _____

Age Identification

Identify the approximate age for each of the following. The erupting teeth are indicated by cross-hatching.

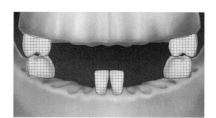

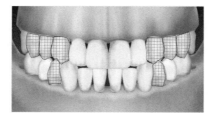

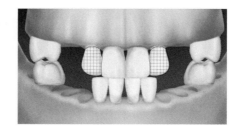

1. _____   2. _____   3. _____

Module **4** Technique Basics

APPLICATION

SELF-ASSESSMENT

Chapters 18 - 24

Based on the worksheets that you have just completed for Chapters 18 - 24, how prepared are you for the upcoming Module 4 assessments?

_____ very prepared, confident

_____ somewhat prepared, somewhat confident

_____ somewhat unprepared, lack confidence

_____ unprepared, no confidence

Based on your answer above, what is your plan for improvement? List the topics and concepts that you need to further review and study for assessments.

_____

_____

_____

_____

_____

_____

_____

CRITICAL THINKING QUESTIONS

What does all the information in Chapters 18 to 24 mean to you in the practice setting? Use the questions below to help you apply the information that you have just learned. Work in pairs and practice answering these questions with your classmates. Share feedback concerning the content and delivery of information—is the information correct and understandable for the average patient? Are effective communication skills being used? The more you practice, the more comfortable you will be discussing these issues with your patients.

1. **After exposing and processing images, the dental radiographer notices that all four of the bite-wing images have overlapped contact areas and cone-cuts. Why did these errors happen, and what can the dental radiographer do to correct them?**

   • CHAPTER 19

2. **After exposing bite-wing images, the dental radiographer notices that neither molar exposure shows the necessary teeth for a diagnostic image. Why did this error happen, and what can the dental radiographer do to correct it?**

   • CHAPTER 19

3. **You are teaching the new dental radiographer in your dental office how to take occlusal images. What is your plan for training her?**

   • CHAPTER 21

4. **A radiopaque object is noted on maxillary molar periapical, superimposed over the roots. Using the buccal object rule, how can you determine whether the object is buccal or lingual?**

   • CHAPTER 21

5. **A 28-year-old woman came to the office for a panoramic image. All procedural steps were followed for panoramic exposure, but upon processing, the image showed a large radiopaque area concealing a portion of the mandible. What caused this error? What must be done in the future to prevent it?**

   • CHAPTER 22

6. **A 22-year-old man came into the office with pain in the jaw joint. He complained about discomfort in both ears and about having trouble opening and closing his mouth. The patient also said that he hears popping and clicking sounds when he eats. What imaging procedure is recommended for this type of issue?**

   • CHAPTER 23

7. **A patient comes into the office for a dental examination. He is hearing impaired and is in a wheelchair. Dental images must be taken today, and the dental radiographer is worried about a communication barrier and how the images can be taken while the patient is in his wheelchair. The patient has come to the office without a caregiver but can read lips. How should the dental radiographer handle this situation?**

   • CHAPTER 24

8. **Your next patient is a boy with Down syndrome. Describe how you will prepare for this patient with special needs, and identify what techniques you can use to make him feel more comfortable and have a positive experience.**

   • CHAPTER 24

TO-DO CHECKLIST

Written Exercises

_____ Complete all worksheets.

_____ Complete bite-wing technique assessment exercises.

_____ Complete buccal object rule exercises.

_____ Complete self-assessment.

Active Learning Experiences

_____ In laboratory, assemble bite-wing RINN devices.

_____ Demonstrate proper placement of receptor in the bite-wing RINN device.

_____ Using a typodont, demonstrate placement of premolar and molar bite-wings with RINN device.

_____ In laboratory, demonstrate bite-wing tab placement on size 2 receptor.

_____ Using a typodont, demonstrate placement of premolar and molar bite-wings with tabs.

_____ Review and answer the critical thinking questions.

_____ Practice answering critical thinking questions with your classmates and provide feedback.

Clinical Laboratory Activities

_____ Complete activities in Section 2, _Laboratory Manual_ (as assigned by instructor).

Assessments

_____ Complete assessments in Section 2, _Laboratory Manual_ (as assigned by instructor).

BITE-WING TECHNIQUE CHECKLIST

premolar bite-wing

___	**front edge**	in middle of lower canine
___	**premolars**	all visible
___	**occlusal plane**	in middle of film
___	**occlusal plane**	parallel with bottom film edge
___	**horizontal**	correct - if open premolar contacts
___	**vertical**	+ 10 degrees
___	**no cone-cuts**	PID centered over film

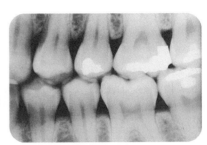

molar bite-wing

___	**front edge**	in middle of lower 2nd premolar
___	**molars**	all visible
___	**occlusal plane**	in middle of film
___	**occlusal plane**	parallel with bottom film edge
___	**horizontal**	correct - if open molar contacts
___	**vertical**	+ 10 degrees
___	**no cone-cuts**	PID centered over film

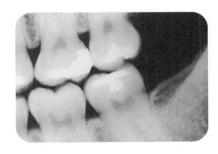

PREMOLAR BITE-WING STEPS

Step 1—Position the PID

- Stand in front of patient.
- Position the PID.

STEPS

1. Place **index finger PARALLEL** to **LOWER PREMOLARS.**

2. Position **open end of PID PARALLEL** with **FINGER.**

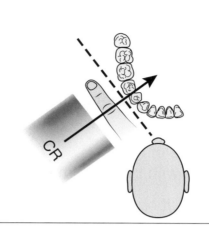

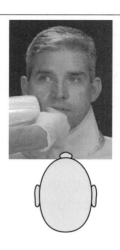

Step 2—Place the Receptor

- Stand in front of patient.
- Place the receptor.

STEPS

1. When placing receptor, **COVER LOWER CANINE** with **front edge.**

2. **HOLD TAB** and instruct patient to **s-l-o-w-l-y close.**

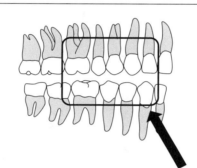

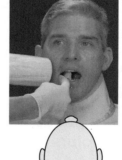

Cover lower canine
with front edge of receptor

Step 3—Check for Cone-cuts

- Stand behind the tubehead.
- Look down PID to check for cone-cut.

STEPS

1. **HOLD TAB** and instruct patient to **smile** to show their teeth.

2. **LOOK DOWN the PID.**

3. If you see the receptor, you will be cone-cut; adjust the PID so you **cannot see the receptor.**

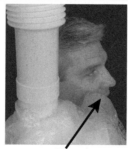

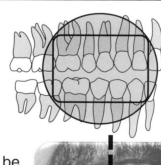

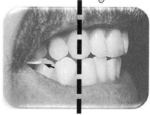

Receptor must be
within diameter of
the PID to avoid a
cone-cut

MOLAR BITE-WING STEPS

Step 1—Position the PID

- Stand in front of patient.
- Position the PID.

STEPS

1. Place **index finger PARALLEL** to **LOWER MOLARS.**

2. Position **open end of PID PARALLEL** with **FINGER.**

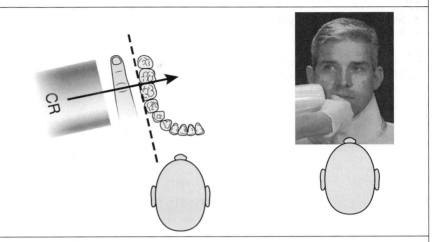

Step 2—Place the Receptor

- Stand in front of patient.
- Place the receptor.

STEPS

1. Place the **FRONT EDGE** in the **middle of the LOWER 2nd PREMOLAR.**

2. **HOLD TAB** and instruct patient to **s-l-o-w-l-y close.**

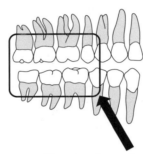

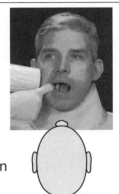

Front edge of receptor placed in middle of lower 2nd premolar

Step 3—Check for Cone-cuts

- Stand behind the tubehead.
- Look down PID to check for cone-cut.

STEPS

1. **HOLD TAB** and instruct patient to **smile** to show their teeth.

2. **LOOK DOWN the PID.**

3. If you see the receptor, you will be cone-cut; adjust the PID so you **cannot see the receptor.**

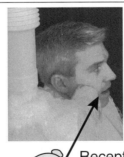

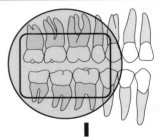

Receptor must be within diameter of the PID to avoid a cone-cut

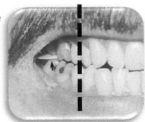

171

OPEN VS. OVERLAPPED CONTACTS

Open Contacts

***CORRECT** horizontal angulation results in **OPEN** contacts.*

For a premolar BW—when the PID opening is PARALLEL to the lower premolars, the horizontal angulation is CORRECT and contacts appear OPEN.

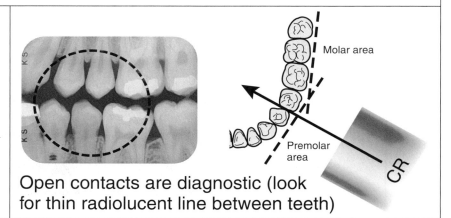

Open contacts are diagnostic (look for thin radiolucent line between teeth)

Overlapped Contacts

***INCORRECT** horizontal angulation results in **OVERLAPPED** contacts.*

For a premolar BW—when the PID opening is NOT PARALLEL to the lower premolars, the horizontal angulation is INCORRECT and contacts appear OVERLAPPED.

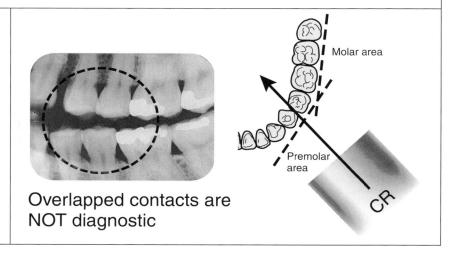

Overlapped contacts are NOT diagnostic

POSITIVE VS. NEGATIVE VERTICAL ANGULATION

A positive vertical angulation (+10 degrees) is used to compensate for the tilt of the maxillary teeth, and if using film or a PSP receptor, the slight bend in upper ½ of receptor.

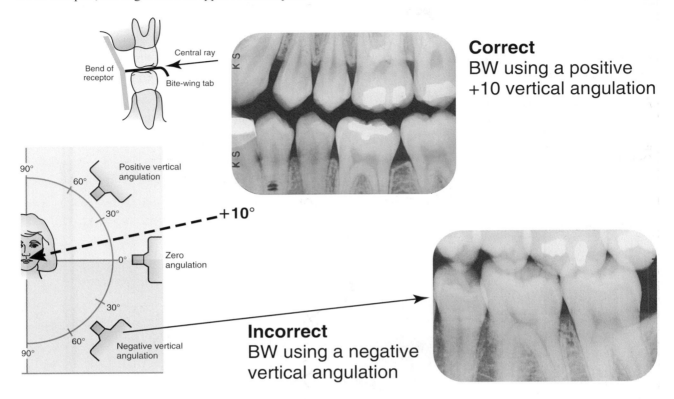

Correct
BW using a positive +10 vertical angulation

Incorrect
BW using a negative vertical angulation

CONE-CUTS

PREMOLAR BITE-WING

To avoid cone-cuts, the PID must be centered over the receptor.

if PID too far back...

if PID too far forward...

cone-cut seen on **front edge**

cone-cut seen on **back edge**

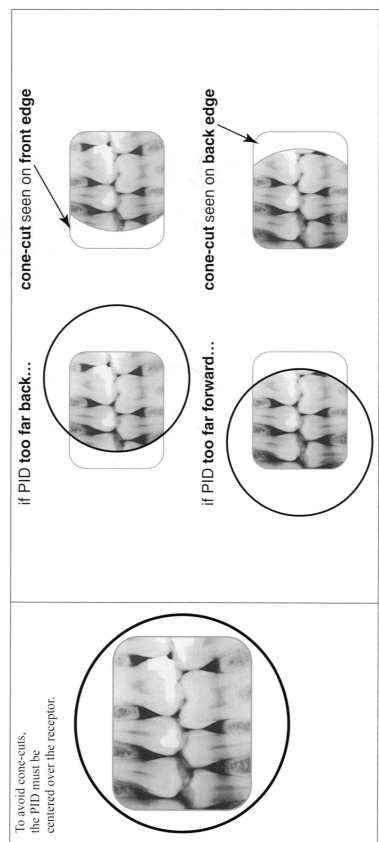

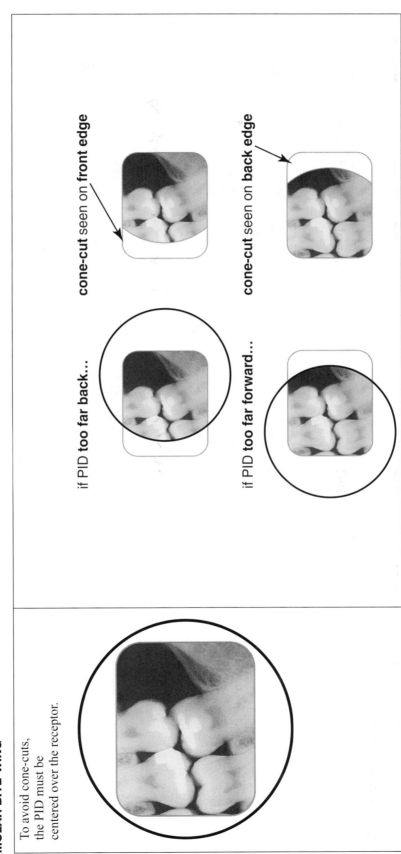

MOLAR BITE-WING

To avoid cone-cuts,
the PID must be
centered over the receptor.

cone-cut seen on **front edge**

cone-cut seen on **back edge**

if PID **too far back**...

if PID **too far forward**...

PANORAMIC PATIENT POSITIONING CHECKLIST

PATIENT PREPARATION

_____ **Explain imaging procedure**

- Briefly explain the imaging procedure to the patient.

_____ **Place lead apron**

- Place and secure a lead apron _without_ a thyroid collar on the patient.

- Place the lead apron low around the neck so that it does not block x-ray beam.

- Use a double-sided lead apron to protect the patient.

_____ **Remove all objects**

- Request that the patient remove all objects from the head-and-neck area that may interfere with the procedure.

- Items to remove include eyeglasses, earrings, intraoral and extraoral piercings, necklaces, napkin chains, hearing aids, hairpins, barrettes, and any intraoral prostheses (complete or partial dentures).

PATIENT POSITIONING

_____ **Position spine**

- Instruct the patient to sit or stand "as tall as possible" with the shoulders back.

- Spine must be perfectly straight.

_____ **Position teeth**

- Instruct the patient to bite in the groove located on the plastic bite block; this aligns the teeth in the focal trough.

- Position maxillary and mandibular anterior in an end-to-end position in the groove on the bite block.

_____ **Position head**

- Position the midsagittal plane (an imaginary plane that divides the patient's face into right and left sides) perpendicular to the floor.

- Position the Frankfort plane (an imaginary plane that passes through the top of the ear canal and the bottom of the eye socket) parallel to the floor.

- Patient's head must not be tipped up or down.

_____ **Position lips and tongue**

- Instruct the patient to place the tongue on the roof of the mouth.

- Suggest that the patient "swallow and feel the tongue rise up to the roof of the mouth" and "keep the tongue in that position during the procedure."

- Instruct the patient to close the lips around the bite block.

_____ **Final instructions and exposure**

- Instruct the patient to remain still while the machine is rotating during exposure.

- Expose the receptor.

MODULE 5 DIGITAL IMAGING BASICS AND NORMAL ANATOMY BASICS

INSTRUCTIONS

How to Prepare
- Review the learning objectives for Module 5 prior to lab.
- Review the critical thinking questions for Module 5 prior to lab.

What to Bring
- *Workbook and Laboratory Manual*—Module 5 materials
- pencil
- textbook (print or e-version)

Written Exercises
- Work together or individually to complete each exercise.
- For each chapter, complete the worksheets in pencil (*without looking up answers*).
- When each exercise is finished, use your text to check answers; correct any wrong answers.
- Use your completed and corrected packet to study for assessments.

Active Learning Experiences
- Using a human skull, identify the normal anatomic features normally viewed on dental images.
- In pairs, take turns answering each critical thinking question and provide feedback to each other.
- Ask your instructor to observe you answering the critical thinking questions and provide you with feedback.

177

5 Digital Imaging Basics and Normal Anatomy Basics

LEARNING OBJECTIVES

The goal of Module 5 laboratory experiences is to provide students with a reinforcement of the fundamental understanding of digital imaging basics, and normal anatomy basics. Upon successful completion of Chapters 25 to 27 lectures and laboratory, the student will be able to:

CHAPTER	LEARNING OBJECTIVES
CHAPTER 25 DIGITAL IMAGING	
Review Text	• Define basic terminology concerning digital imaging. • Describe the basic concepts and purpose of digital imaging. • Describe the equipment needed for digital imaging. • Describe the radiation exposure that occurs with digital imaging. • Describe the different types of sensors used in digital imaging. • Detail the advantages and disadvantages of digital imaging.
CHAPTER 26 THREE-DIMENSIONAL DIGITAL IMAGING	
Review Text	• Define basic terminology concerning three-dimensional digital imaging. • Describe the basic concepts and purpose of three-dimensional digital imaging. • Describe the equipment needed for three-dimensional digital imaging. • Discuss the advantages and disadvantages of three-dimensional digital imaging.
CHAPTER 27 NORMAL ANATOMY: INTRAORAL IMAGES	
Written Exercises	• Define terminology used to describe types of bone, prominences of bone, spaces, and depressions in bone; review the bones of the skull. • Describe the normal anatomic landmarks seen on intraoral images. • Recognize normal anatomic landmarks seen on intraoral images. • Identify the normal anatomy of the maxilla and mandible as radiolucent or radiopaque. • Identify the normal anatomy of the maxilla and mandible as appearing on maxillary images, mandibular images, or both. • Identify normal anatomy of teeth as viewed on intraoral images. • Recognize soft tissue areas identified on intraoral images.
Active Learning Experiences	• On a human skull, identify the normal anatomic structures viewed on intraoral images. • Review the normal anatomy of the maxilla and mandible as viewed on a skull.

WORKBOOK EXERCISES

Chapter 27 Normal Anatomy: Intraoral Images

NORMAL ANATOMY CROSSWORD PUZZLE 1

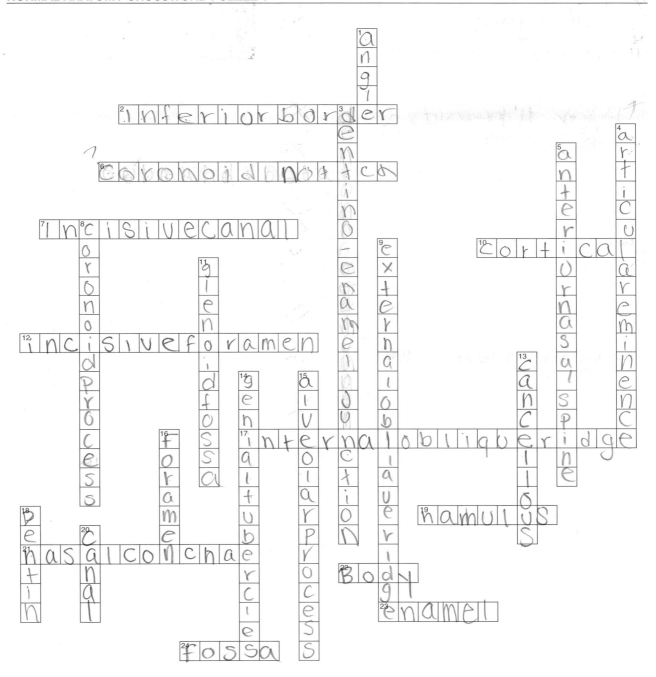

ACROSS

2 a linear prominence of cortical bone that defines the lower border of the mandible

6 a scooped-out concavity of bone located distal to the coronoid process on the ramus of the mandible

7 a passageway through bone that extends from the superior foramina of the incisive canal to the incisive foramen

10 the dense outer layer of bone; appears radiopaque

12 a hole in bone located at the midline of the anterior portion of the hard palate directly posterior to the maxillary central incisors; appears radiolucent

17 a linear prominence of bone located on the internal surface of the mandible that extends downward and forward from the ramus; appears radiopaque

19 a small, hooklike process of bone that extends from the medial pterygoid plate of the sphenoid bone; appears radiopaque

21 wafer-thin, curved plates of bone that extend from the lateral walls of the nasal cavity and appear radiopaque

22 the horizontal, U-shaped portion of mandible that extends from ramus to ramus

23 the densest structure found in the human body; the outermost radiopaque layer of the crown of a tooth

24 a broad, shallow, scooped-out, or depressed area of bone; appears radiolucent

DOWN

1 area of the mandible where the body meets the ramus

3 the junction between the dentin and enamel of a tooth

4 a rounded projection of the temporal bone located anterior to the glenoid fossa

5 a sharp projection of the maxilla located at the anteroinferior portion of the nasal cavity; appears radiopaque

8 a marked prominence of bone located on the anterior ramus of the mandible; appears radiopaque

9 a linear prominence of bone located on the external surface of the body of the mandible; appears radiopaque

11 a concave, depressed area of the temporal bone where the mandibular condyle rests

13 the soft, spongy bone located between two layers of dense cortical bone; appears radiolucent

14 tiny bumps of bone located on the lingual anterior mandible; serve as attachment sites for muscles; appear radiopaque

15 portion of the mandible that encases and supports teeth

16 an opening or hole in bone that permits the passage of nerves and blood vessels; appears radiolucent

18 the tooth layer found beneath the enamel and surrounding the pulp cavity; appears radiopaque

20 a tubelike passageway through bone that houses nerves and blood vessels; appears radiolucent

Name Kelsey Rubin

Date

NORMAL ANATOMY CROSSWORD PUZZLE 2

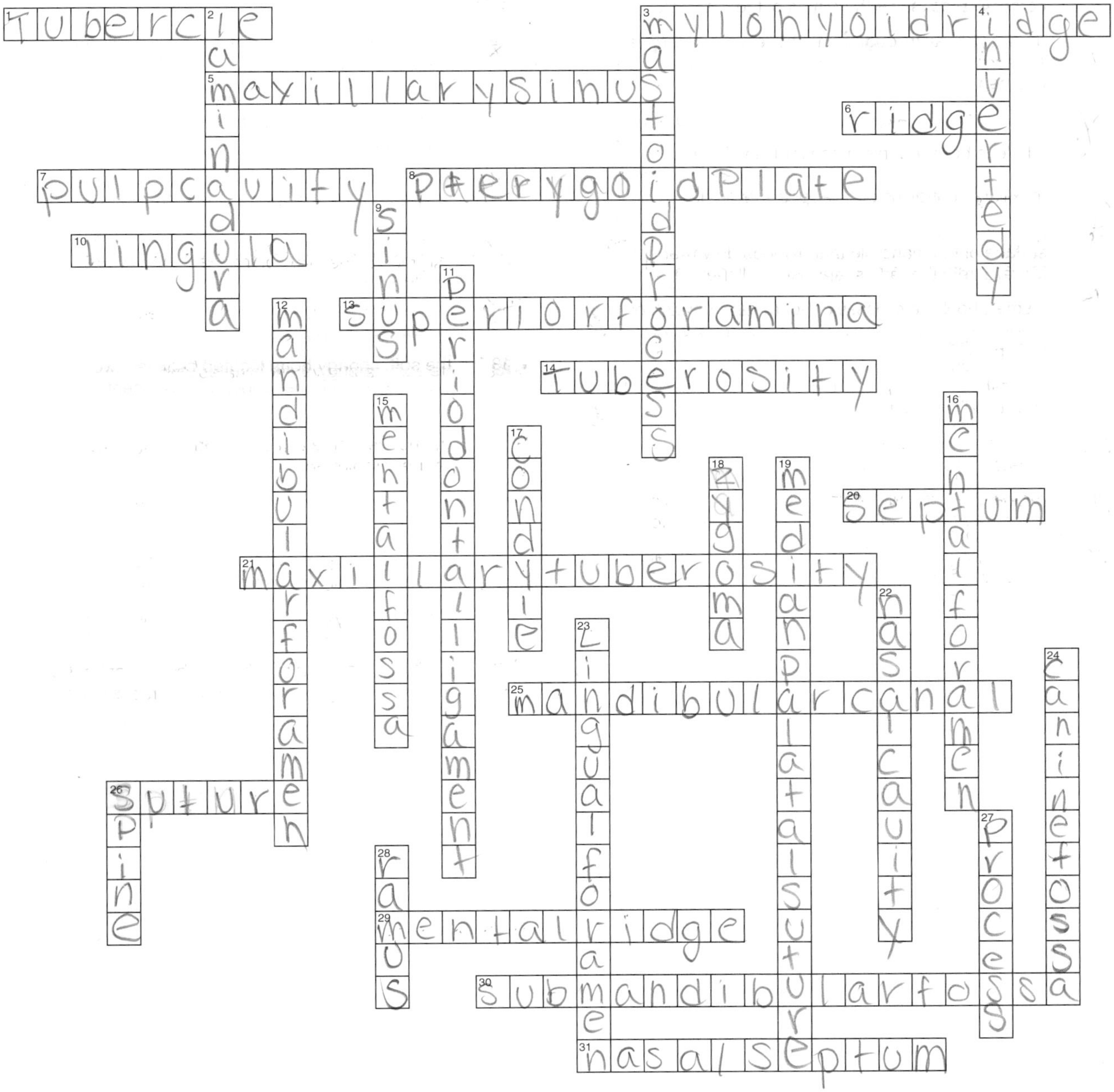
1 Tubercle
2 lamina dura
3 mylohyoid ridge
3 mastoid process
4 inverted Y
5 maxillary sinus
6 ridge
7 pulp cavity
8 pterygoid plate
9 sinus
10 lingula
11 periodontal ligament
12 mandibular foramen
13 superior foramina
14 Tuberosity
15 mental fossa
16 mental foramen
17 condyle
18 zygoma
19 median palatal suture
20 septum
21 maxillary tuberosity
22 nasal cavity
23 lingual foramen
24 canine fossa
25 mandibular canal
26 suture
26 spine
27 process
28 ramus
29 mental ridge
30 submandibular fossa
31 nasal septum

ACROSS

1. a small bump or nodule of bone; appears radiopaque

3. a linear prominence of bone located on the internal surface of the mandible that extends from the molar region downward and forward; appears radiopaque

5. a compartment of bone located within the maxilla and located superior to the posterior teeth; appears radiolucent

6. a linear prominence or projection of bone; appears radiopaque

7. a cavity within a tooth that contains blood vessels, nerves, and lymphatics; appears radiolucent

8. a wing-shaped bony projection of the sphenoid bone located distal to the maxillary tuberosity region

10. a small, tongue-shaped projection of bone seen adjacent to the mandibular foramen

13. two tiny holes in bone that are located on the floor of the nasal cavity at the opening of the incisive canal; appears radiolucent

14. a rounded prominence of bone; appears radiopaque

20. Bony wall that divides a cavity into separate areas; appears radiopaque

21. a rounded prominence of bone that extends posterior to the third molar region; appears radiopaque

25. a tubelike passageway through bone that travels the length of the mandible; appears radiolucent

26. an immovable joint that represents a line of union between adjoining bones of the skull; appears radiolucent

29. a linear prominence of cortical bone located on the external surface of the anterior portion of the mandible; appears radiopaque

30. a depressed area of bone located on the internal surface of the mandible inferior to the mylohyoid ridge; appears radiolucent

31. a vertical bony wall or partition that divides the nasal cavity; appears radiopaque

DOWN

2. the wall of the tooth socket that surrounds the root of a tooth; appears radiopaque

3. a marked prominence of bone located distal to the temporomandibular joint

4. a radiographic landmark that represents the intersection of the maxillary sinus and the nasal cavity; appears radiopaque

9. a hollow space, cavity, or recess in bone; appears radiolucent

11. a space that exists between the root of a tooth and the lamina dura; contains connective tissue fibers, blood vessels, and lymphatics; appears radiolucent

12. a round or ovoid hole in bone on the lingual aspect of the ramus of the mandible

15. a scooped-out, depressed area of bone located on the external surface of the anterior mandible; appears radiolucent

16. an opening or hole in bone located on the external surface of the mandible in the premolar region; appears radiolucent

17. a rounded projection of bone extending from the posterosuperior border of the ramus of the mandible

18. the bone that appears as a diffuse radiopaque band posterior to the zygomatic process of the maxilla

19. the immovable joint between the two palatine processes of the maxilla; appears radiolucent

22. a pear-shaped compartment of bone located superior to the maxilla; appears radiolucent

23. an opening or hole in bone located on the internal surface of the mandible near the midline; surrounded by genial tubercles and appears radiolucent

24. a smooth, depressed area of the maxilla located adjacent to the canine; appears radiolucent

26. a sharp, thornlike projection of bone; appears radiopaque

27. a marked prominence or projection of bone; appears radiopaque

28. vertical portion of the mandible that is found posterior to the third molar

IDENTIFICATION

Identify each item as radiolucent or radiopaque. Place a check mark (✔) in the appropriate column.

Radiolucent	Radiopaque		Radiolucent	Radiopaque	
General Terms			**Bony Landmarks of Mandible**		
✔		1 canal		✔	32 coronoid process
	✔	2 canal—borders of		✔	33 external oblique ridge
	✔	3 cortical bone		✔	34 genial tubercles
✔		4 foramen		✔	35 inferior border of mandible
✔		5 fossa		✔	36 internal oblique ridge
	✔	6 process	✔		37 lingual foramen
	✔	7 ridge	✔		38 mandibular canal
	✔	8 septum	✔		39 mental foramen
✔		9 sinus	✔		40 mental fossa
	✔	10 spine		✔	41 mental ridge
✔		11 suture		✔	42 mylohyoid ridge
	✔	12 tubercle	✔		43 nutrient canals
	✔	13 tuberosity	✔		44 submandibular fossa
Bony Landmarks of Maxilla			**Normal Tooth Anatomy**		
	✔	14 anterior nasal spine		✔	45 alveolar crest—anterior
	✔	15 hamular process		✔	46 alveolar crest—posterior
✔		16 incisive foramen		✔	47 dentin
	✔	17 inferior nasal conchae		✔	48 dentino-enamel junction
	✔	18 inverted Y		✔	49 enamel
✔		19 lateral fossa		✔	50 lamina dura
✔		20 maxillary sinus	✔		51 periodontal ligament space
	✔	21 maxillary sinus floor	✔		52 pulp cavity
✔		22 maxillary sinus nutrient canals	**Soft Tissue**		
✔		23 maxillary sinus septa	✔		53 lip line
	✔	24 maxillary tuberosity		✔	54 nasolabial groove
✔		25 median palatal suture	✔		55 nose
✔		26 nasal cavity			
	✔	27 nasal cavity floor			
	✔	28 nasal septum			
✔		29 superior foramina of incisive canal			
	✔	30 zygoma			
	✔	31 zygomatic process of maxilla			

Name Kelsey Rubin
Date _____

Identify each item listed as appearing on a maxillary image, a mandibular image, or on both. Place a check mark (✔) in the appropriate column or columns.

Kelsey Rubin

	Found on Maxillary Images	Found on Mandibular Images	Item
1	✓	✓	alveolar crest
2	✓		anterior nasal spine
3	✓		coronoid process
4		✓	external oblique ridge
5		✓	genial tubercles
6	✓		hamular process
7	✓		incisive foramen
8		✓	inferior border of mandible
9	✓		inferior nasal conchae
10	✓		internal oblique ridge
11	✓		inverted Y
12	✓	✓	lamina dura
13	✓		lateral fossa
14		✓	lingual foramen
15		✓	mandibular canal
16	✓		maxillary sinus
17	✓		maxillary sinus floor
18	✓		maxillary sinus nutrient canals
19	✓		maxillary sinus septa
20	✓		maxillary tuberosity
21	✓		median palatal suture
22		✓	mental foramen
23		✓	mental fossa
24		✓	mental ridge
25		✓	mylohyoid ridge
26	✓		nasal cavity
27	✓		nasal cavity floor
28	✓		nasal septum
29	✓		nasolabial groove
30	✓		nose outline
31	✓	✓	nutrient canals
32			periodontal ligament space
33	✓	✓	submandibular fossa
34	✓		superior foramina of incisive canal
35	✓		zygoma
36	✓		zygomatic process of maxilla

Identify each structure in Fig. 27-1.

1. maxillary tuberosity
2. coronoid process
3. nasal cavity
4. nasal septum
5. anterior nasal spine
6. external oblique ridge
7. mental foramen
8. mental ridge
9. mental fossa

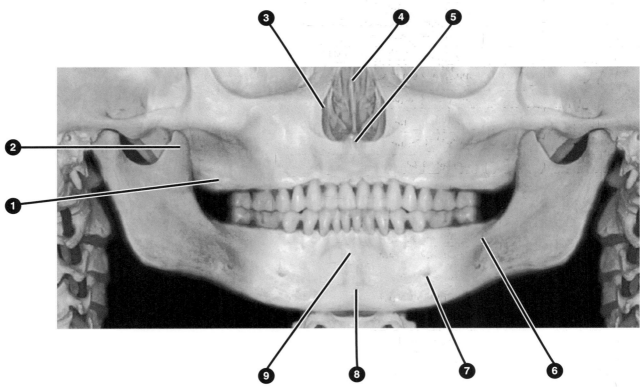

Fig. 27-1 From White SC, Pharoah MJ: [*Oral radiology*] *principles and interpretation*, ed 7, St. Louis, 2014, Mosby.

Module **5** **Digital Imaging Basics and Normal Anatomy Basics**

Kelsey Rubin

Identify each structure in Fig. 27-2.

1. enamel
2. Dentino-enamel junction
3. Dentin
4. pulp cavity
5. Periodontal ligament space
6. lamina dura
7. alveolar crest
   crest of alveolar ridge

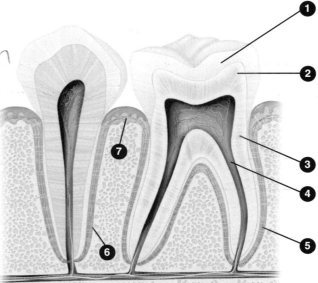

Fig. 27-2

Identify each structure in Fig. 27-3.

8. internal oblique ridge
9. submandibular fossa
10. mylohyoid ridge
11. genial tubercles

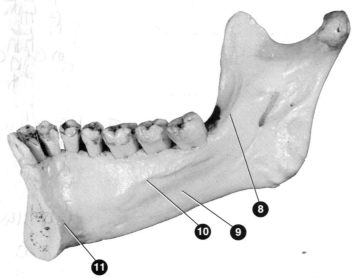

Fig. 27-3 From Liebgott B: _The anatomic basis of dentistry,_ ed 3, St. Louis, 2011, Mosby.

Identify each structure in Fig. 27-4.

1. _maxilla_te_____

2. _inferior nasal conchae_____

3. _palatine bone_____

?4. _medical pterygoid plate_____

5. _hamular process_____

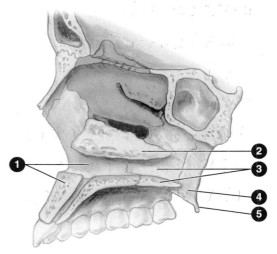

Fig. 27-4 From Fehrenbach and Herring: *Illustrated anatomy of the head and neck,* ed 4, St. Louis, 2011, Saunders.

Identify each structure in Fig. 27-5.

6. _corohoid process_____

7. _alveolar process_____

8. _inferior border of mah__

9. _mental fossa_____

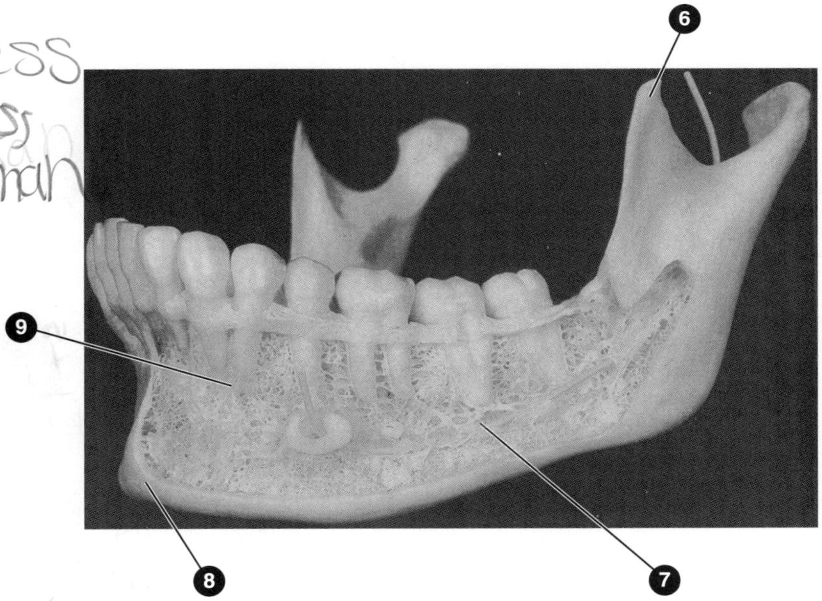

Fig. 27-5 From Logan BM, Reynold PA, Hutching RT: *McMinn's color atlas of head and neck anatomy,* ed 4, London, 2010, Mosby Ltd.

Module 5 **Digital Imaging Basics and Normal Anatomy Basics**

Kelsey Rubin

Identify each structure in Fig. 27-6.

1. Inferior nasal conchae
2. Zygoma
3. Zygomatic process of maxilla
4. External oblique ridge
5. Mental foramen
6. Mental ridge
7. Max tuberosity
8. Anterior nasal spine
9. Nasal septum

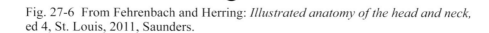

Fig. 27-6 From Fehrenbach and Herring: *Illustrated anatomy of the head and neck,* ed 4, St. Louis, 2011, Saunders.

Kelsey Rubin

LABELING EXERCISE

Draw an arrow from each numbered item to the correct area on *both* the skull photo and the intraoral image.

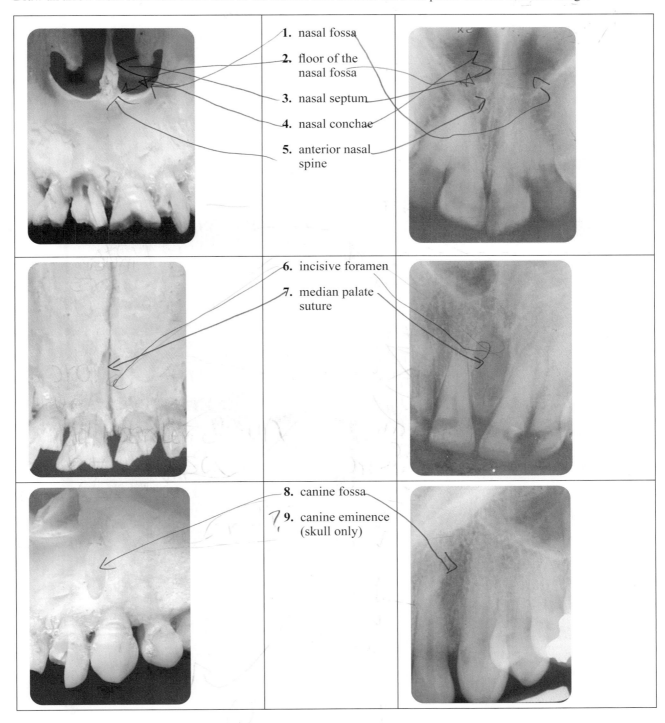

1. nasal fossa
2. floor of the nasal fossa
3. nasal septum
4. nasal conchae
5. anterior nasal spine

6. incisive foramen
7. median palate suture

8. canine fossa
9. canine eminence (skull only)

189

Kelsey Rubin

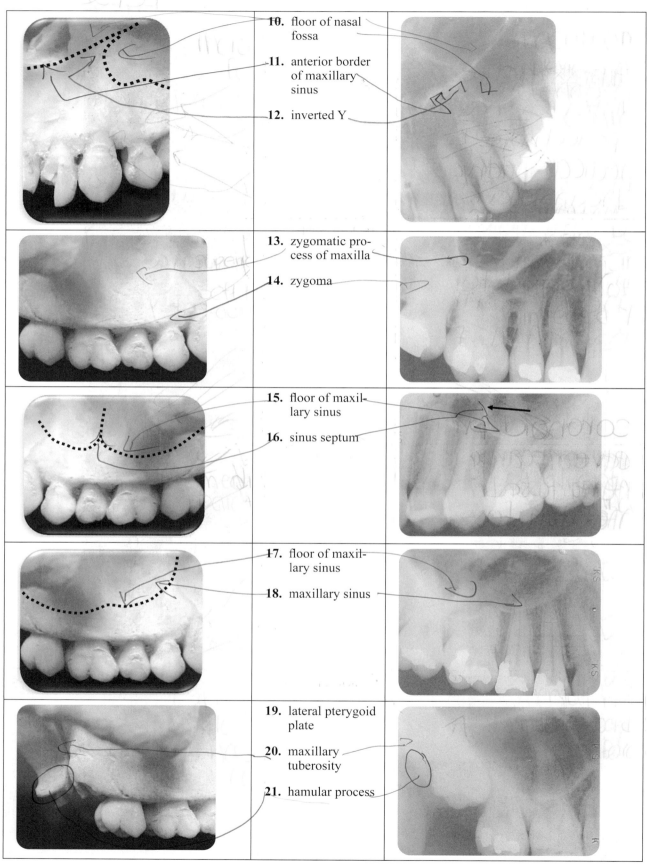

10. floor of nasal fossa

11. anterior border of maxillary sinus

12. inverted Y

13. zygomatic process of maxilla

14. zygoma

15. floor of maxillary sinus

16. sinus septum

17. floor of maxillary sinus

18. maxillary sinus

19. lateral pterygoid plate

20. maxillary tuberosity

21. hamular process

Kelsey Rubin

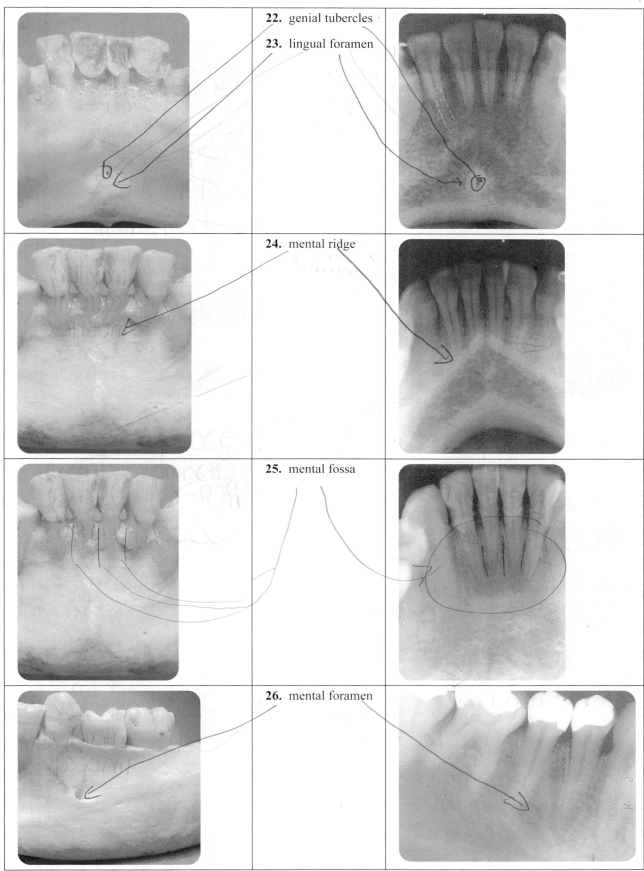

22. genial tubercles
23. lingual foramen
24. mental ridge
25. mental fossa
26. mental foramen

191

Kelsey Rubin

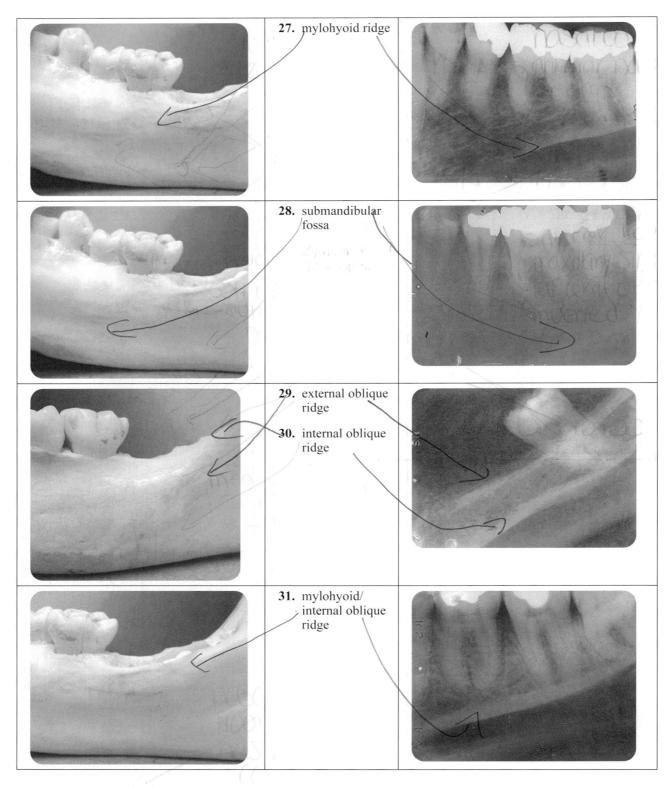

27. mylohyoid ridge

28. submandibular fossa

29. external oblique ridge

30. internal oblique ridge

31. mylohyoid/ internal oblique ridge

Kelsey Rubin

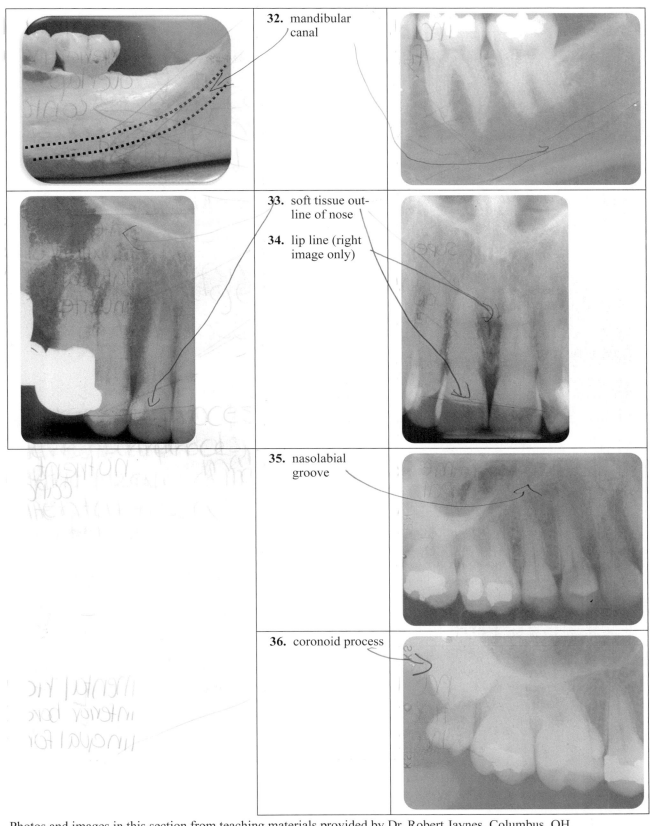

32. mandibular canal

33. soft tissue outline of nose

34. lip line (right image only)

35. nasolabial groove

36. coronoid process

Photos and images in this section from teaching materials provided by Dr. Robert Jaynes, Columbus, OH.

193

Identify each of the numbered structures.

Kelsey Rubin

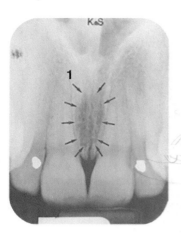

1. incisive foramen

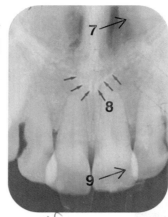

7. nasal conchae
8. anterior nasal spine
9. overlap contact

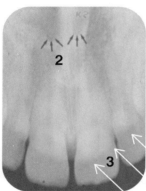

2. superior foramina of incisive canal
3. soft tissue outline of nose

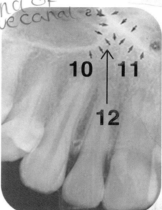

anterior border of
10. maxillary sinus
11. lat wall of nasal fossa
12. inverted Y

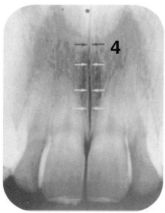

4. median palatal suture

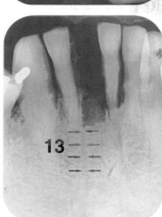

13. nutrient canal

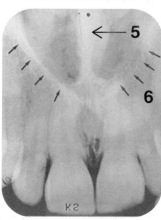

5. nasal septum
6. floor of nasal cavity

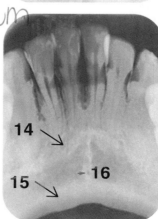

14. mental ridge
15. inferior border of man
16. lingual foramen

Kelsey Rubin

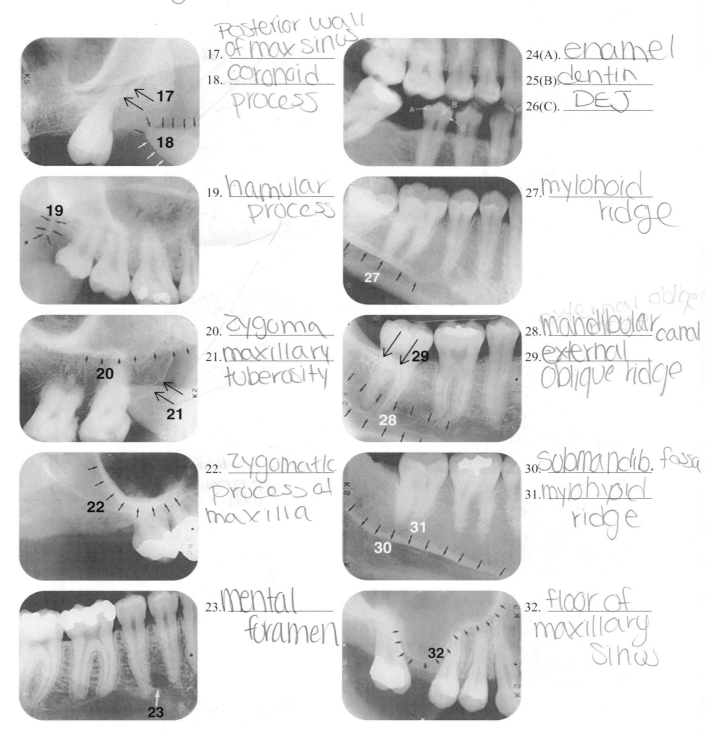

17. Posterior wall of max sinus
18. coronoid process

24(A). enamel
25(B). dentin
26(C). DEJ

19. hamular process

27. mylohoid ridge

20. zygoma
21. maxillary tuberosity

28. mandibular canal
29. external oblique ridge

22. zygomatic process of maxilla

30. submandib. fossa
31. mylohyoid ridge

23. mental foramen

32. floor of maxillary sinus

Images in this section from teaching materials provided by Dr. Robert Jaynes, Columbus, OH.

✗ stop ✗

APPLICATION

Module 5 Digital Imaging Basics and Normal Anatomy Basics

SELF-ASSESSMENT

Chapters 25 - 27

Based on the worksheets that you have just completed for Chapters 25 - 27, how prepared are you for the upcoming assessments?

_____ very prepared, confident

_____ somewhat prepared, somewhat confident

_____ somewhat unprepared, lack confidence

_____ unprepared, no confidence

Based on your answer above, what is your plan for improvement? List the topics and concepts that you need to further review and study for assessments.

_____

_____

_____

_____

_____

_____

CRITICAL THINKING QUESTIONS

What does all the information in Chapters 25 to 27 mean to you in the practice setting? Use the questions below to help you apply the information that you have just learned. Work in pairs and practice answering these questions with your classmates. Share feedback concerning the content and delivery of information—is the information correct and understandable for the average patient? Are effective communication skills being used? The more you practice, the more comfortable you will be discussing these issues with your patients.

1. **If you were helping to plan a new practice, which type of imaging system (digital versus film based) would you choose and why?**

    • CHAPTER 25

2. **A patient in your office needs to be referred for three-dimensional imaging in order to begin her implant treatment planning. How will you explain the importance of obtaining three-dimensional imaging in terms that the patient can understand?**

    • CHAPTER 26

3. **Why is it important for dental professionals to learn about the anatomy of the skull? Give examples of how knowledge of normal anatomy is needed in everyday practice.**

    • CHAPTER 27

TO-DO CHECKLIST

Written Exercises

_____ Complete all worksheets.

_____ Complete self-assessment.

Active Learning Experiences

_____ Complete all normal anatomy exercises.

_____ Using a human skull, identify the normal anatomic features normally viewed on dental images.

_____ Review and answer the critical thinking questions.

_____ Practice answering critical thinking questions with your classmates and provide feedback.

RADIOLUCENT AND RADIOPAQUE REVIEW

RADIOLUCENT

- air space
- foramen
- canal
- suture
- fossa
- pdl space

- soft tissue

- cancellous bone

- cortical bone
- lamina dura
- dentin
- enamel

- metal restorations

RADIOPAQUE

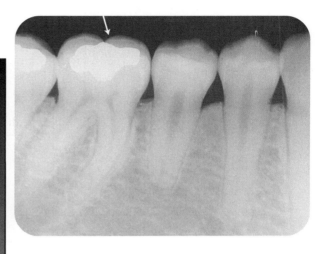

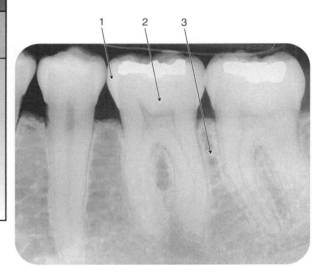

Normal Anatomy on Intraoral Images

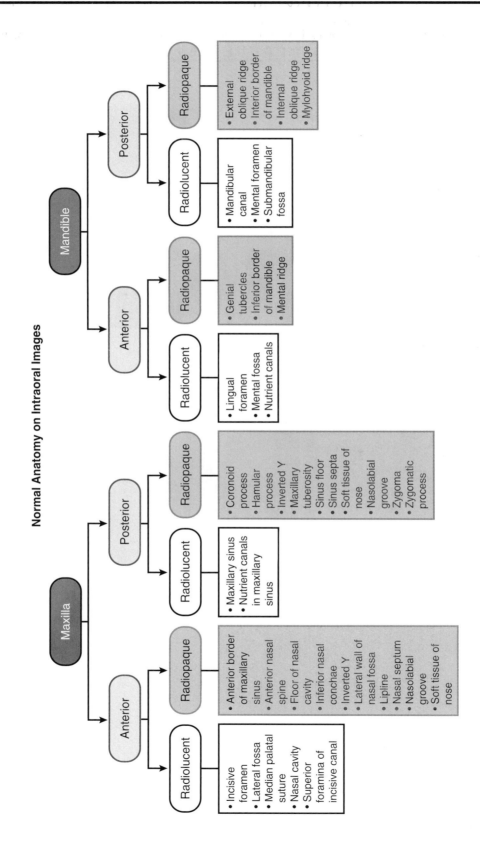

Maxilla

Anterior

Radiolucent
- Incisive foramen
- Lateral fossa
- Median palatal suture
- Nasal cavity
- Superior foramina of incisive canal

Radiopaque
- Anterior border of maxillary sinus
- Anterior nasal spine
- Floor of nasal cavity
- Inferior nasal conchae
- Inverted Y
- Lateral wall of nasal fossa
- Lipline
- Nasal septum
- Nasolabial groove
- Soft tissue of nose

Posterior

Radiolucent
- Maxillary sinus
- Nutrient canals in maxillary sinus

Radiopaque
- Coronoid process
- Hamular process
- Inverted Y
- Maxillary tuberosity
- Sinus floor
- Sinus septa
- Soft tissue of nose
- Nasolabial groove
- Zygoma
- Zygomatic process

Mandible

Anterior

Radiolucent
- Lingual foramen
- Mental fossa
- Nutrient canals

Radiopaque
- Genial tubercles
- Inferior border of mandible
- Mental ridge

Posterior

Radiolucent
- Mandibular canal
- Mental foramen
- Submandibular fossa

Radiopaque
- External oblique ridge
- Interior border of mandible
- Internal oblique ridge
- Mylohyoid ridge

BONES REVIEW

On the following pages, you will find a review of some of the bones of the skull. Included is a variety of skull views to help you picture what goes where. This material may be used to supplement your existing anatomy materials.

- SPHENOID

- ETHMOID

- VOMER

- PALATINE BONES

- ZYGOMATIC BONE

- MAXILLA

- MANDIBLE

SPHENOID BONE

OVERVIEW

- single bone

- located at midline of cranium

- articulates with frontal, parietal, ethmoid, temporal, zygomatic, maxillary, palatine, vomer, and occipital bones

- connects cranial skeleton to facial skeleton

- resembles a bat with extended wings

- complex, very difficult to visualize

LANDMARKS

Foramina and Fissures

- carry important nerves and blood vessels

- **superior orbital fissure** (CN V, ophthalmic)

- **foramen ovale** (CN V, mandibular), **foramen rotundum** (CN V, maxillary) and **foramen spinosum**

Body

- middle portion of the sphenoid

- articulates anteriorly with ethmoid

- articulates posteriorly with occipital

- contains paired **sphenoidal sinuses**

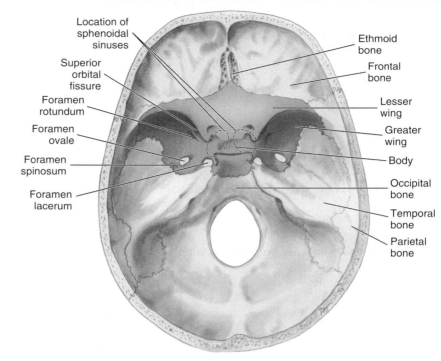

From Fehrenbach and Herring. *Illustrated anatomy of the head and neck*, ed 4, St. Louis, 2011, Saunders.

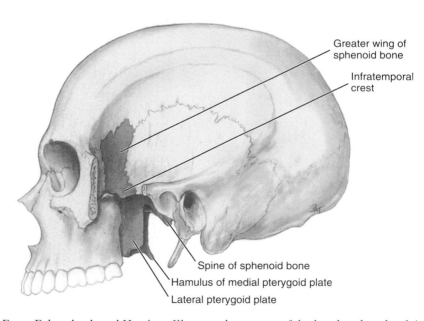

From Fehrenbach and Herring. *Illustrated anatomy of the head and neck*, ed 4, St. Louis, 2011, Saunders.

Processes

- **three paired processes**—lesser wing, greater wing. and pterygoid process

- **lesser wing** is anterior

- **greater wing** is posterolateral

- **pterygoid process**

  - inferior to greater wing

  - attachment site for muscles of mastication

  - consists of two plates: **lateral and medial pterygoid plates**

  - **pterygoid fossa** is in between pterygoid plates

  - **hamulus**, a hooklike projection of bone, extends from medial pterygoid plate

- **sphenoidal spine**

  - sharp, pointed area at posterior corner of greater wing

- **infratemporal crest**

  - divides the greater wing into two smaller surfaces

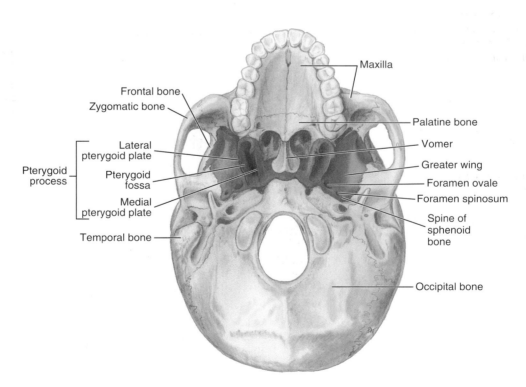

From Fehrenbach and Herring. *Illustrated anatomy of the head and neck*, ed 4, St. Louis, 2011, Saunders.

203

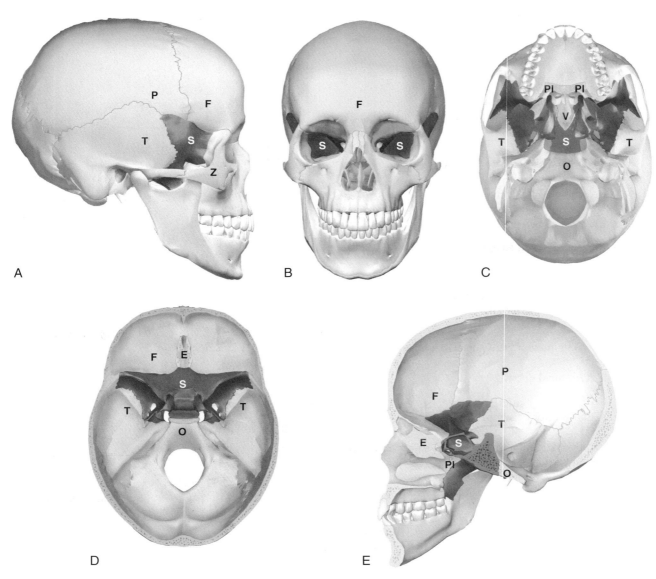

From Liebgott B. *The anatomical basis of dentistry*, ed 3, St. Louis, 2011, Mosby.

ETHMOID BONE

OVERVIEW

- single bone

- located at midline

- articulates with frontal, sphenoid, lacrimal, and maxillary bones

- connects cranial skeleton to facial skeleton

- difficult to visualize (like sphenoid bone)

LANDMARKS

Plates and Associated Structures

- ethmoid has two unpaired plates

- **perpendicular plate** is vertical, **cribriform plate** is horizontal

- **perpendicular plate**

  o seen in nasal cavity

  o joins vomer at inferior and posterior borders

  o with vomer and nasal septal cartilage, forms **nasal septum**

- **crista galli** is the vertical continuation of the perpendicular plate into cranial cavity

- **cribriform plate**

  o is visible inside the cranial cavity

  o present on superior aspect

  o perforated by foramina to allow passage of olfactory nerves for smell

Nasal Conchae and Associated Structures

- **nasal conchae**

  o lateral portions form **superior and middle nasal conchae** in nasal cavity

- **orbital plate**

  o forms medial wall of orbit

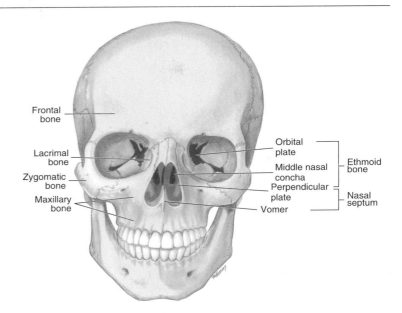

Frontal bone · Lacrimal bone · Zygomatic bone · Maxillary bone · Orbital plate · Middle nasal concha · Perpendicular plate · Vomer · Ethmoid bone · Nasal septum

From Fehrenbach and Herring. *Illustrated anatomy of the head and neck*, ed 4, St. Louis, 2011, Saunders.

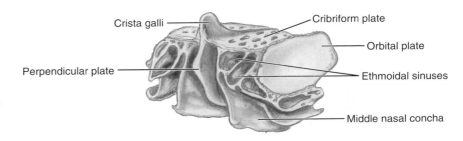

Crista galli · Perpendicular plate · Cribriform plate · Orbital plate · Ethmoidal sinuses · Middle nasal concha

From Fehrenbach and Herring. *Illustrated anatomy of the head and neck*, ed 4, St. Louis, 2011, Saunders.

- **ethmoidal sinuses**

  ○ found between orbital plate and conchae

  ○ consist of air-filled spaces

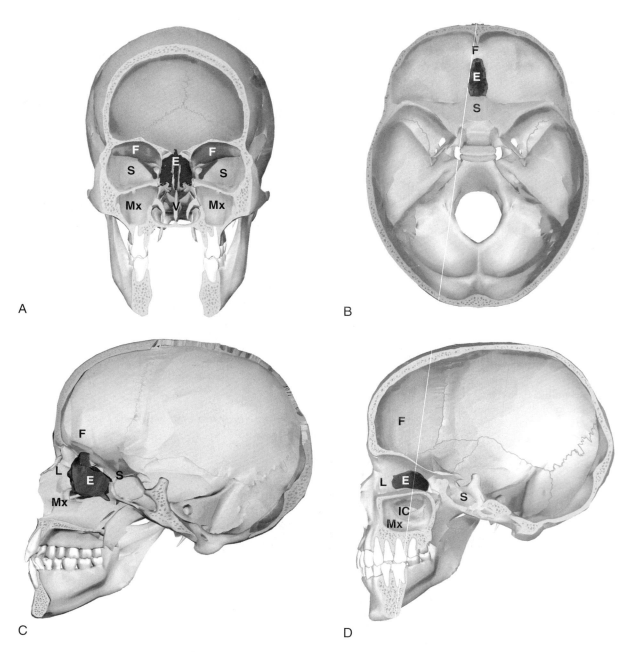

From Liebgott B. *The anatomical basis of dentistry*, ed 3, St. Louis, 2011, Mosby.

VOMER

OVERVIEW

- single facial bone

- located at midline

- forms posterior nasal septum[1]

- articulates with

    - ethmoid

    - nasal cartilage

    - palatine bones

    - maxilla

    - sphenoid bone

- posteroinferior border is free—no bony articulation

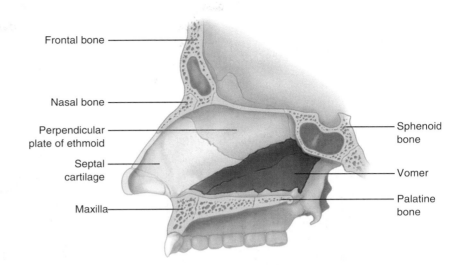

Fonseca R, Barber DH, Powers M, Frost DE. *Oral and maxillofacial trauma*, ed 4, St. Louis, 2013, Saunders.

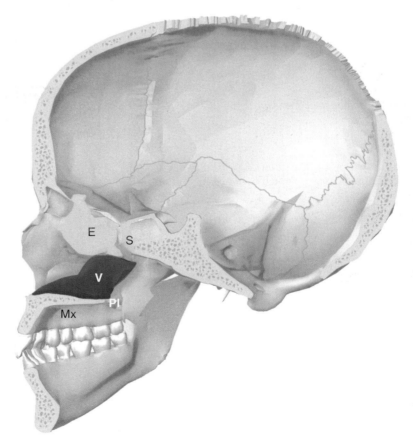

From Liebgott B. *The anatomical basis of dentistry*, ed 3, St. Louis, 2011, Mosby.

---

[1] nasal septum formed by the perpendicular plate of the ethmoid, the vomer, and nasal cartilage

207

PALATINE BONES

OVERVIEW

- paired bones of skull

- form parts of nasal cavity, oral cavity, pterygopalatine fossa, and orbit

- articulates with maxilla, sphenoid, ethmoid, vomer, inferior concha, and opposite palatine bone

- shaped like an *L* and joins its counterpart as a mirror image

- has a vertical and horizontal (palatal) portion

LANDMARKS

Plates

- **horizontal plates**

  - form posterior 1/3 of hard palate

  - posterior border is smooth and concave

  - horizontal plates articulate with each other at posterior portion of **median palatine suture**

- **vertical plates** form a portion of lateral walls of nasal cavity

  - **medial/nasal surface**

  - **roughened lateral surface** articulates with maxilla

  - vertical plate has three processes

  - superior aspect has two processes: anterior **orbital process** and posterior **sphenoidal process,** separated by a notch; **sphenoidal notch** separates the two processes

Foramina

- transmit nerves and blood vessels to this region

- **greater palatine foramen**

  - located in posterolateral area

  - near apex of maxillary third molar

  - transmits greater palatine nerve and blood vessels

  - landmark for administration of greater palatine local anesthetic block

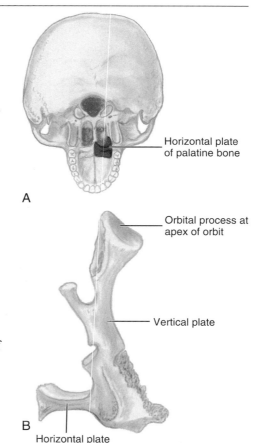

Horizontal plate of palatine bone

A

Orbital process at apex of orbit

Vertical plate

B

Horizontal plate

From Fehrenbach and Herring. *Illustrated anatomy of the head and neck*, ed 4, St. Louis, 2011, Saunders.

- **lesser palatine foramen**

  o smaller opening

  o transmits the **lesser palatine nerve** and blood vessels to soft palate and tonsils

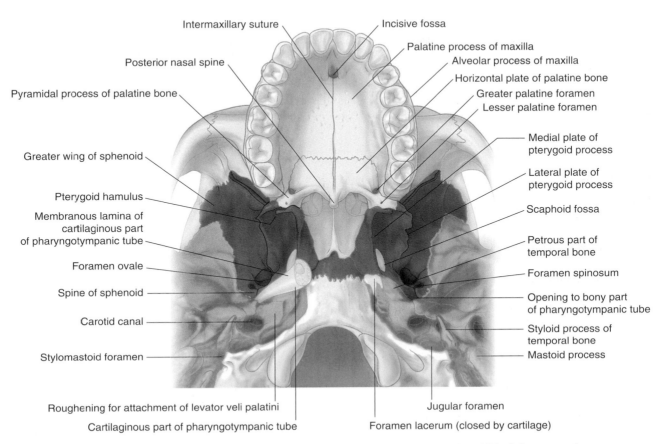

From Drake, RL. *Gray's anatomy for students*, 3e, London, 2015, Churchill Livingstone.

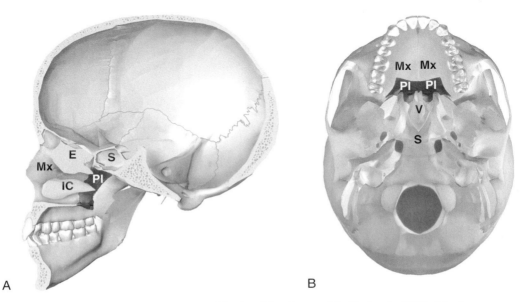

From Liebgott B *The anatomical basis of dentistry*, ed 3, St. Louis, 2011, Mosby.

ZYGOMATIC BONE (ZYGOMA)

OVERVIEW

- paired bones of face

- forms cheekbones

- forms zygomatic arch, lateral wall of orbit, and anterior wall of infratemporal region

- articulates with frontal bone, greater wing of the sphenoid, maxilla, and temporal bone

LANDMARKS

PROCESSES

- **frontal process** articulates superiorly with frontal bone

- **maxillary process** articulates with the maxilla inferiorly

- **temporal process** articulates posteriorly with the zygomatic process of the temporal bone

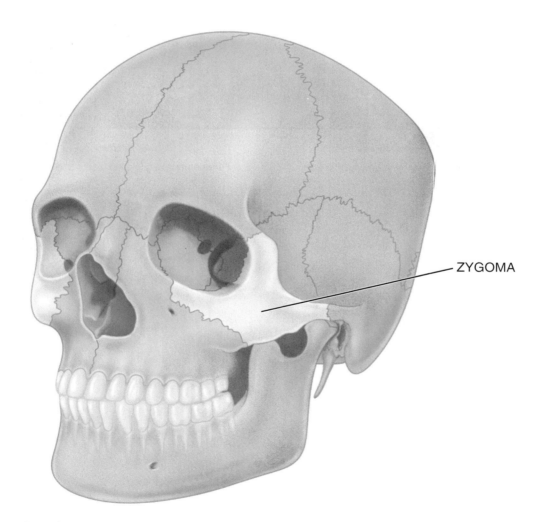

ZYGOMA

Fonseca R, Barber DH, Powers M, Frost DE. *Oral and maxillofacial trauma*, ed 4, St. Louis, 2013, Saunders.

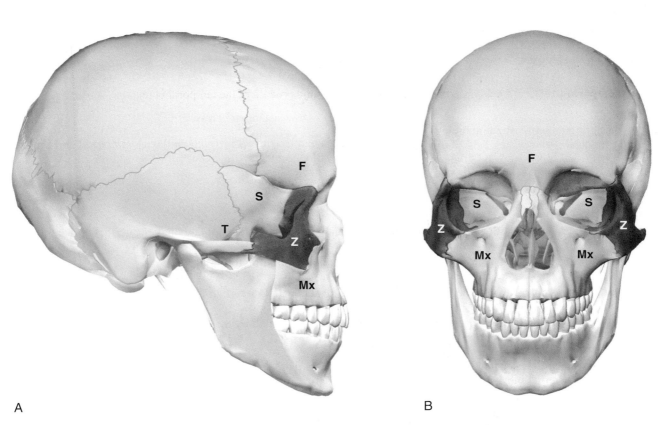

A

B

From Liebgott B. *The anatomical basis of dentistry*, ed 3, St. Louis, 2011, Mosby.

Module **5** **Digital Imaging Basics and Normal Anatomy Basics**

MAXILLAE

OVERVIEW

- paired maxillary bones

- fused at intermaxillary suture

- together form the upper jaw

- articulate with frontal, lacrimal, nasal, inferior nasal conchae, vomer, sphenoid, ethmoid, palatine, and zygomatic bones

- each maxilla includes a body and **four processes**: frontal, zygomatic, palatine, and alveolar

LANDMARKS

Body

- has orbital, nasal, infratemporal, and facial surfaces

- contains air-filled spaces called maxillary sinuses

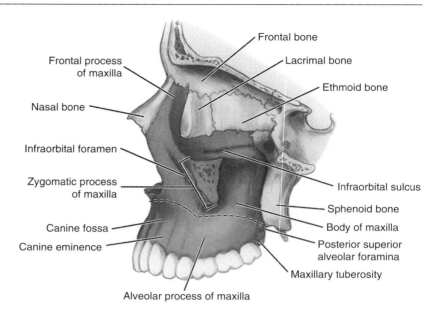

From Fehrenbach and Herring. *Illustrated anatomy of the head and neck*, ed 4, St. Louis, 2011, Saunders.

Processes

- **frontal**: articulates with frontal bone and forms medial orbital rim with lacrimal bone on anterior surface

- **zygomatic**: articulates with zygoma laterally and completes infraorbital rim

- **palatine**: articulates with other maxilla bone via the median palatal suture to form anterior hard palate

- **alveolar**: horseshoe-shaped area of bone that encases roots of maxillary teeth

Other Structures

- **incisive foramen**: located at the anterior midline between the palatine processes of the maxillae and posterior to maxillary central incisors; carries right and left nasopalatine nerves and blood vessels from nasal cavity to anterior hard palate

- **canine fossa:** elongated depression just posterior and superior to the root of the maxillary canine

- **canine eminence:** prominent facial ridge over the maxillary canine

- **maxillary tuberosity**: rounded prominence of bone on the posterior part of the body of the maxilla, just posterior to the most distal molar of the maxillary arch

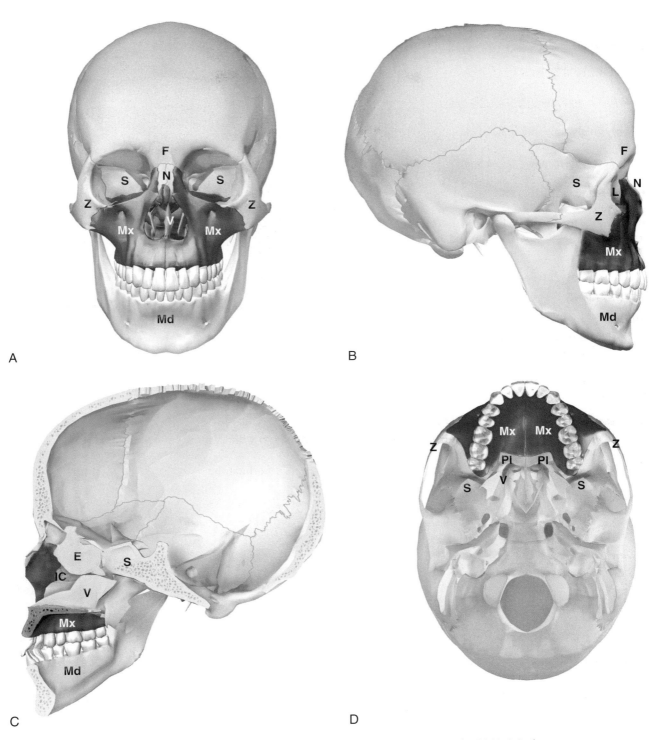

From Liebgott B. *The anatomical basis of dentistry*, ed 3, St. Louis, 2011, Mosby.

MANDIBLE

OVERVIEW

- single facial bone

- forms lower jaw

- only freely movable bone of skull

- largest and strongest facial bone

- horseshoe shaped

- movable articulation with temporal bones at each temporomandibular joint

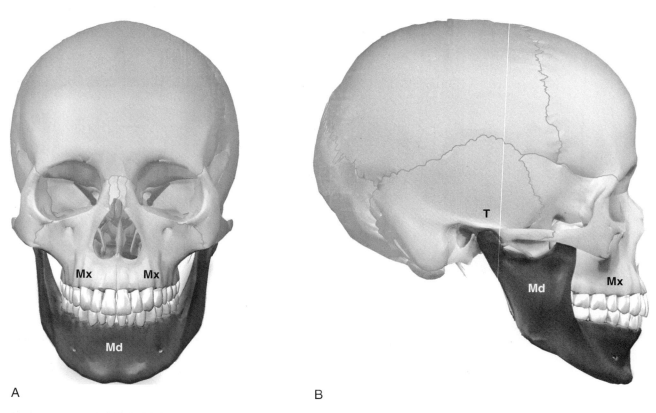

A

B

From Liebgott B. *The anatomical basis of dentistry*, ed 3, St. Louis, 2011, Mosby.

LANDMARKS

Anterior View

- **mental protuberance**: bony prominence of the chin, located below the roots of mandibular incisors

- **mandibular symphysis**: faint ridge at the midline on the anterior surface where the bone is formed by the fusion of right and left processes during development

- **mental foramen**: hole in bone located inferior to the apices of the mandibular first and second premolars; allows the passage of the mental nerve and blood vessels

- **body**: the heavy horizontal part inferior to the mental foramen, lateral view

Lateral View

- **ramus**: on the lateral aspect of the mandible, the flat plate that extends superiorly and posteriorly from the body of the mandible

- **angle**: where the body of the mandible meets the ramus

- **coronoid notch**: main part of the anterior border of the ramus forms a concave forward curve; this greatest depression on the anterior border of the ramus is a landmark for administration of IA block

- **external oblique line**: a ridge inferior to the coronoid notch where the anterior border of the ramus joins the body of the mandible

- **coronoid process**: anterior border of the ramus is a thin, sharp margin that terminates in triangular shaped area of bone

- **condyloid process**: consists of mandibular condyle and the neck (constricted part that supports it)

- **condyle**: ovoid prominence of bone that is found on posterior-superior border of ramus

- **mandibular notch** or **sigmoid notch**: depression between the coronoid process and condyle

Medial View

- **genial tubercles**: tiny bumps of bone near the midline that serve as muscle attachments

- **retromolar triangle**: area at the lateral edge of each mandibular alveolar process, just posterior to the last molar

- **internal oblique ridge/mylohyoid line**: along each medial surface is a ridge that extends posteriorly and superiorly, becoming more prominent as it ascends

- **submandibular fossa**: a depressed area below the posterior part of the mylohyoid line and inferior to the mandibular posterior teeth

- **mandibular foramen**: opening of mandibular canal on the medial surface of the ramus; inferior alveolar nerve and blood vessels enter the mandible via this foramen

- **lingual**: a thin flap of bone overhanging the mandibular foramen; serves as an attachment site for sphenomandibular ligament

To make flashcards, cut along solid lines and fold in half at the dashed line.

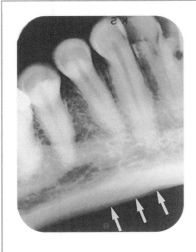

identify this **radiopaque** band

inferior border of the mandible

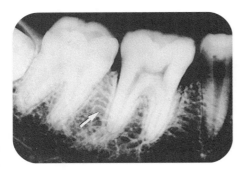

identify this **type of bone**

cancellous bone

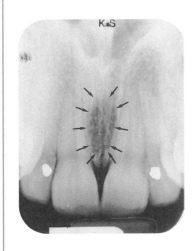

identify this ovoid **radiolucency**

incisive foramen

Module **5** **Digital Imaging Basics and Normal Anatomy Basics**

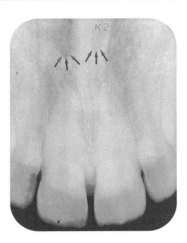

identify the **radiolucent** areas

superior foramina
of incisive canal

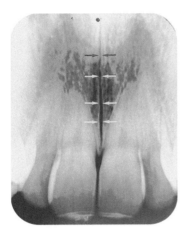

identify the thin **radiolucent** line

median palatal suture

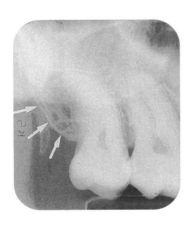

identify the **radiopaque** area

maxillary tuberosity

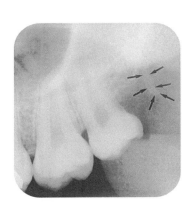

identify the
radiopaque
area

hamulus
(hamular process)

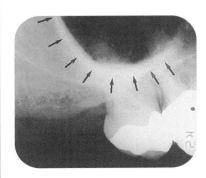

identify the
radiopaque
area

**zygomatic
process**
of maxilla

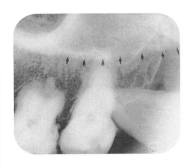

identify the
radiopaque
band

zygoma

Module **5** Digital Imaging Basics and Normal Anatomy Basics

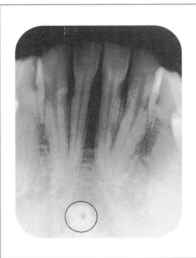

identify the round **radiopacity**

genial tubercles

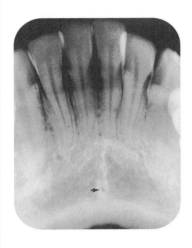

identify the **radiolucent** dot

lingual foramen

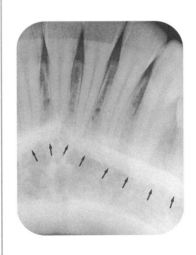

identify this **radiopaque** band

mental ridge

Module **5** Digital Imaging Basics and Normal Anatomy Basics

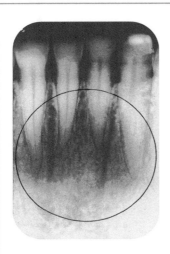 identify this **radiolucent** area	**mental fossa**
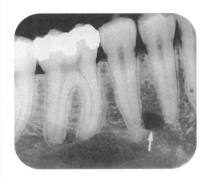 identify this **radiolucency**	**mental foramen**
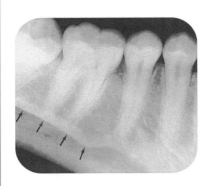 identify this **radiopaque** band	**mylohyoid ridge**

Module **5**   **Digital Imaging Basics and Normal Anatomy Basics**

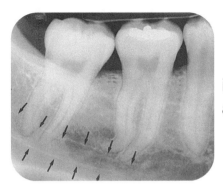

identify this area

mandibular canal

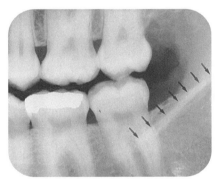

identify this **radiopaque** band

external oblique ridge

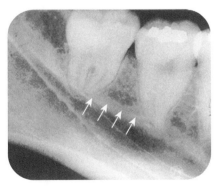

identify this **radiopaque** band

internal oblique ridge

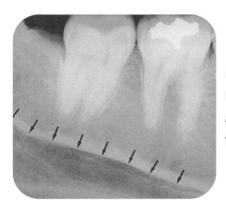

identify the **radiolucent** area below the arrows

submandibular fossa

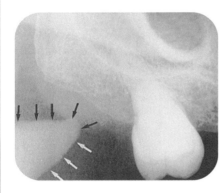

identify this **radiopacity**

coronoid process

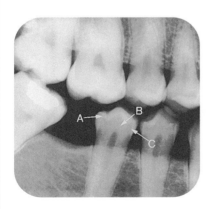

identify a, b, & c

a - enamel
b- dentin
c- DEJ

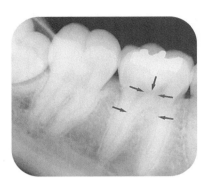

identify the **radiolucent** areas

pulp chamber & pulp canals

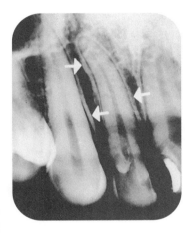

identify the **radiopaque** areas

lamina dura

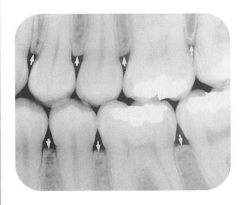

identify this area of bone

crestal lamina dura

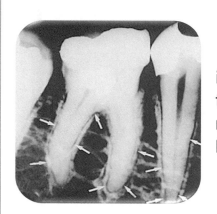

identify the thin **radiolucent** line

periodontal ligament space

MODULE **6** FILM MOUNTING, NORMAL ANATOMY, AND INTERPRETATION BASICS

INSTRUCTIONS

How to Prepare
- Review the learning objectives for Module 6 prior to lab.
- Review the critical thinking questions for Module 6 prior to lab.

What to Bring
- *Workbook and Laboratory Manual*—Module 6 materials
- pencil
- textbook (print or e-version)

Written Exercises
- Work together or individually to complete each exercise.
- For each chapter, complete the worksheets in pencil (*without looking up answers*).
- When each exercise is finished, use your text to check answers; correct any wrong answers.
- Use your completed and corrected packet to study for assessments.

Active Learning Experiences
- Using the Interactive Exercises on Evolve, practice mounting digital images.
- Practice mounting a complete series of films (if available).
- Using a human skull, identify anatomic features normally viewed on a panoramic image.
- In pairs, take turns answering each critical thinking question and provide feedback to each other.
- Ask your instructor to observe you answering the critical thinking questions and provide you with feedback.

6

Film Mounting, Normal Anatomy, and Interpretation Basics

LEARNING OBJECTIVES

The goal of Module 6 laboratory experiences is to provide students with a reinforcement of the fundamental understanding of film mounting, normal anatomy, and interpretation basics. Upon successful completion of Chapters 28 to 31 lectures and laboratory, the student will be able to:

CHAPTER	LEARNING OBJECTIVES
CHAPTER 28 FILM MOUNTING AND VIEWING	
Written Exercises	• Practice mounting a complete series of dental images using a labeled template.
Active Learning Experiences	• Using the Interactive Exercises on Evolve, practice mounting digital images.
	• If films and mounts are available, practice mounting a complete series of dental films.
	• Check each other's mounted films for accuracy.
	• Mount a complete series in 5 minutes or less.
CHAPTER 29 NORMAL ANATOMY: PANORAMIC IMAGES	
Written Exercises	• Identify normal findings (anatomic features, air spaces, and soft tissue shadows) on a panoramic image.
	• Review the six areas of a diagnostic panoramic image.
	• Identify and describe the normal anatomic landmarks of the maxilla as viewed on a panoramic image.
	• Identify and describe the normal anatomic landmarks of the mandible as viewed on a panoramic image.
	• Identify and describe the appearance of air spaces as viewed on a panoramic image.
	• Identify and describe the appearance of soft tissue as viewed on a panoramic image.
Active Learning Experiences	• Identify and describe the normal anatomic landmarks of the maxilla on a human skull.
	• Identify and describe the normal anatomic landmarks of the mandible on a human skull.
	• Complete an interpretation worksheet for each panoramic image provided.
CHAPTER 30 INTRODUCTION TO INTERPRETATION	
Written Exercises	• Define the roles of the dentist and dental auxiliary in the interpretation of dental images.
	• Describe who is able to interpret dental images.
	• Summarize the importance of the interpretation of images.
	• Discuss the difference between interpretation and diagnosis.
	• Describe when and where dental images are interpreted.
	• Describe how image interpretation can be used to educate the dental patient about the importance and use of dental images.
CHAPTER 31 DESCRIPTIVE TERMINOLOGY	
Written Exercises	• Describe lesions on a dental image in terms of appearance, location, and size.

Name Kelsey Rubin

Date 9-28-20

WORKBOOK EXERCISES

Chapter 28 Film Mounting and Viewing

IMAGE MOUNTING EXERCISES

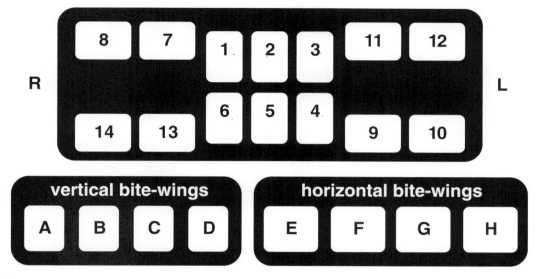

Using the labeled templates above, identify where each of the following images should be mounted. Please note that some images may appear upside down. Use normal anatomic landmarks to help you orient each image.

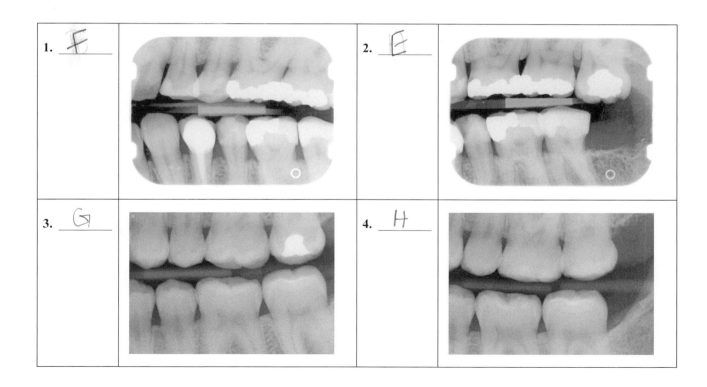

1. F

2. E

3. G

4. H

Module **6** Film Mounting, Normal Anatomy, and Interpretation Basics

Kelsey Rubin

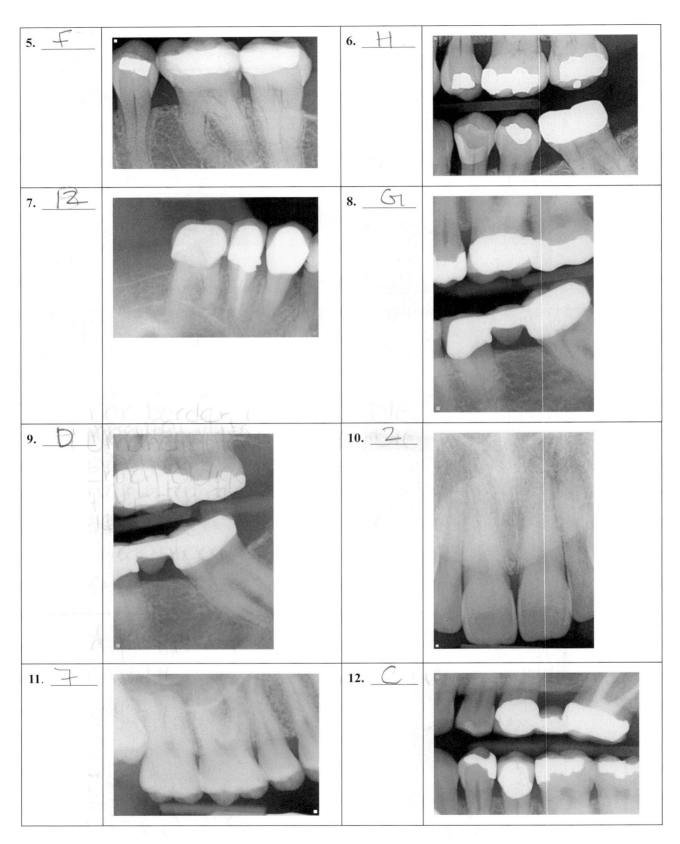

5. F

6. H

7. 13

8. G

9. D

10. 2

11. 7

12. C

13. B

14. H

15. 7

16. 10

17. 12

18. 6

19. B

20. 12

Module 6 Film Mounting, Normal Anatomy, and Interpretation Basics

Kelsey Rubin

21. 13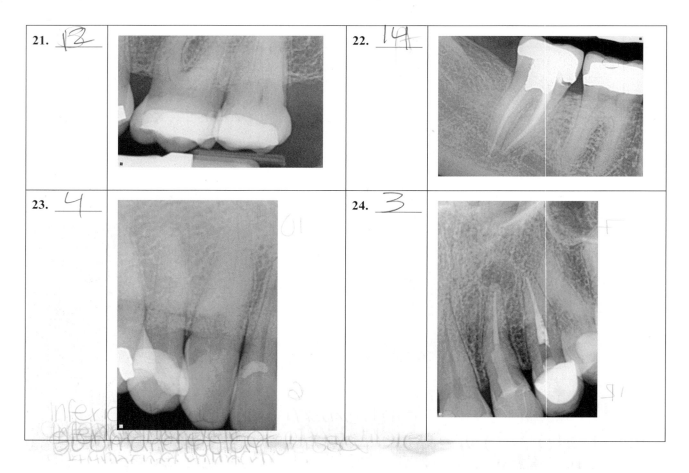

22. 14

23. 4

24. 3

inferior

WORKBOOK EXERCISES

Chapter 29   Normal Anatomy: Panoramic Images

IDENTIFICATION

As you complete the following exercises, when viewing a panoramic image, picture the skull as illustrated below.

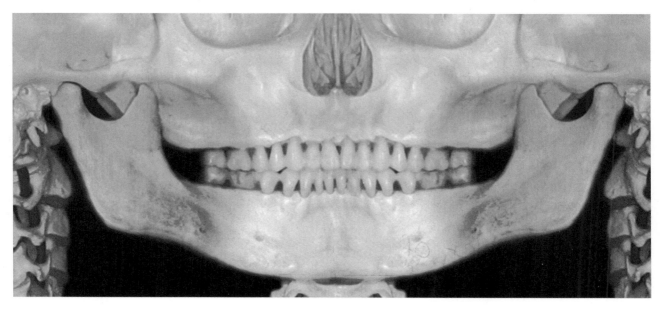

From White SC, Pharoah MJ. *Oral radiology: principles and interpretation*, ed 7, St. Louis, Mosby, 2014.

Module **6   Film Mounting, Normal Anatomy, and Interpretation Basics**

Kelsey Rubin

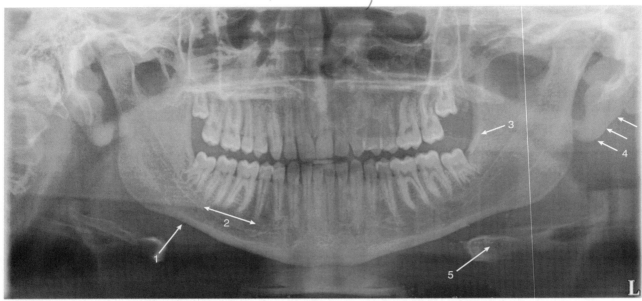

Fig. 29-1

Normal Anatomic Landmarks

Identify each area labeled 1 to 5 in Fig. 29-1.

1. Inferior border of mandible
2. Submandibular fossa
3. external oblique ridge
4. Soft tissue of ear
5. hyoid bone

Name Kelsey Rubin

Date _____

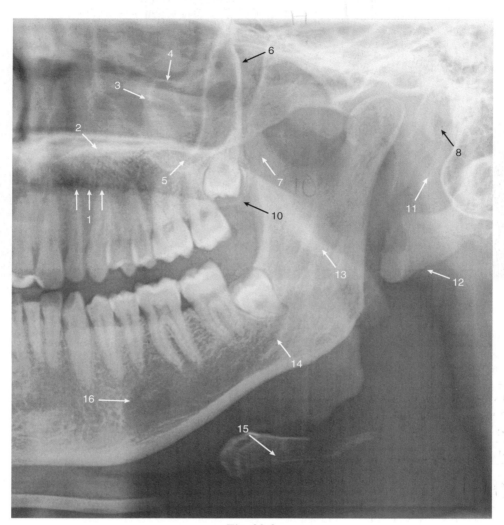

Fig. 29-2

Identify each area labeled 1 to 16 in Fig. 29-2.

1. incisive foramen
2. hard palate
3. maxillary tuberosity
4. maxillary sinus
5. maxillary sinus
6. Posterior wall of max. sinus
7. hamulus
8. unsure

9. not listed ?????
10. maxillary tuberosity
11. styloid process
12. soft tissue of ear
13. mandibular foramen
14. mandibular canal
15. hyoid bone
16. mental foramen

243

Kelsey Rubin

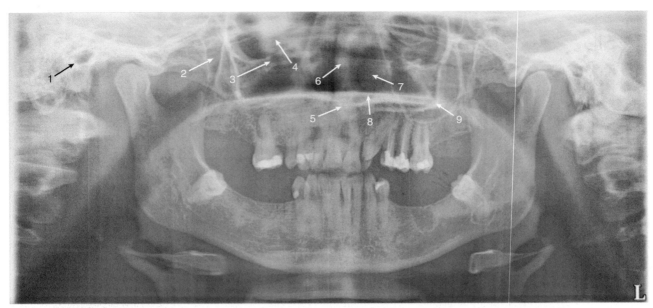

Fig. 29-3

Identify each area labeled 1 to 9 in Fig. 29-3.

1. external auditory meatus
2. pterygomaxillary fissure
3. infraorbital foramen
4. orbit
5. anterior nasal spine
6. nasal septum
7. nasal conchae
8. hard palate
9. zygomatic process of maxilla

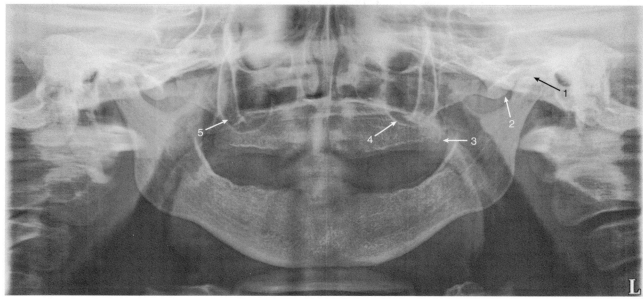

Fig. 29-4

Identify each area labeled 1 to 5 in Fig. 29-4.

1. Glenoid fossa

2. Articular eminence

3. Maxillary tuberosity

4. Maxillary sinus

5. zygoma

Kelsey Rubin

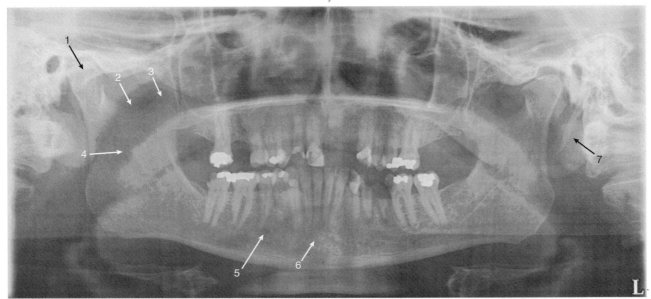

Fig. 29-5

Identify each area labeled 1 to 7 in Fig. 29-5.

1. condyle
2. sigmoid notch
3. coronid process
4. mandibular foramen
5. mental foramen
6. genial tubercle
7. styloid process

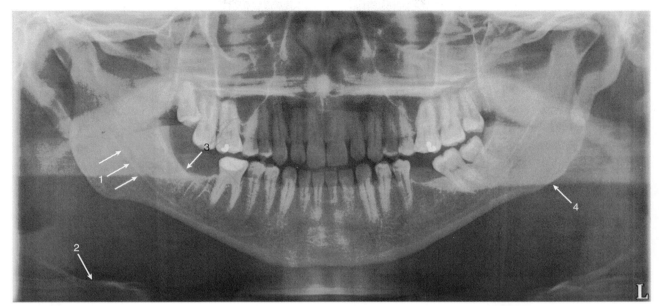

Fig. 29-6

Identify each area labeled 1 to 4 in Fig. 29-6.

1. mandibular canal
2. hyoid bone
3. internal oblique ridge
4. angle of mandible

Kelsey Rubin

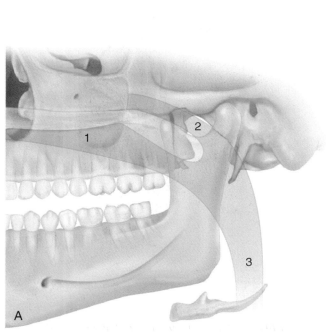

Fig. 29-7A

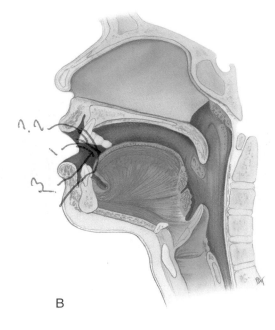

B

Fig. 29-7B From Fehrenbach and Herring.
Illustrated anatomy of the head and neck, ed 4, St.
Louis, 2011, Saunders.

Air Spaces and Soft Tissue

Label **air spaces** 1 to 3 in Fig. 29-7A. Then draw arrows to identify the **air spaces** 1 to 3 on the diagram in Fig. 29-7B.

1. palatoglossal airspace
2. nasopharyngeal air space
3. glossopharyngeal air space

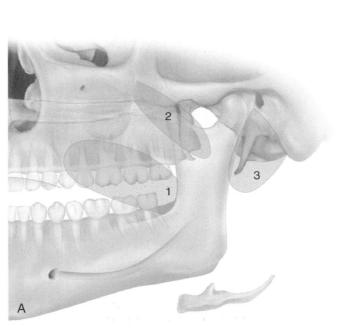

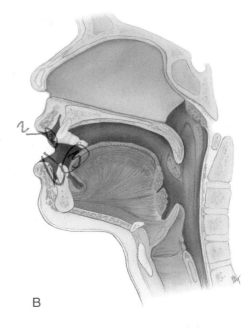

A

Fig. 29-8A

B

Fig. 29-8B From Fehrenbach and Herring.
Illustrated anatomy of the head and neck, ed 4, St.
Louis, 2011, Saunders.

Label **soft tissue areas** 1 to 3 in Fig. 29-8A. Then draw arrows to identify the **soft tissue areas** 1 to 3 on the diagram in Fig. 29-8B.

1. tongue

2. soft palate + uvula

3. lipline

Kelsey Rubin

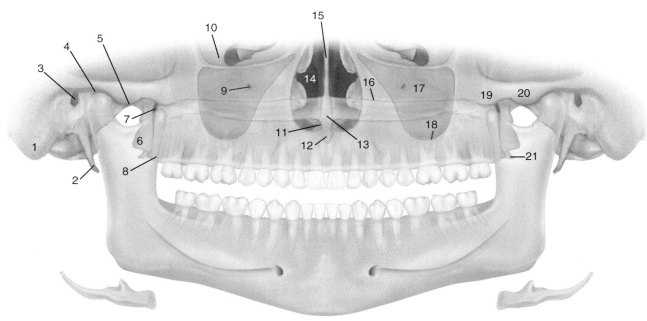

Fig. 29-9

Normal Anatomy of Maxilla

Identify each structure labeled 1 to 21 in Fig. 29-9.

1. mastoid process
2. styloid process
3. external auditory meatus
4. glenoid fossa
5. articular eminence
6. lateral pterygoid plate
7. pterygomaxillary fissure
8. maxillary tuberosity
9. infraorbital foramen
10. orbit

11. incisive canal
12. incisive foramen
13. anterior nasal spine
14. nasal cavity + conchae
15. nasal septum
16. hard palate
17. maxillary sinus
18. floor of maxillary sinus
19. zygomatic process of maxilla
20. zygomatic arch
21. hamulus

Name _Kelsey Rubin_

Date _____

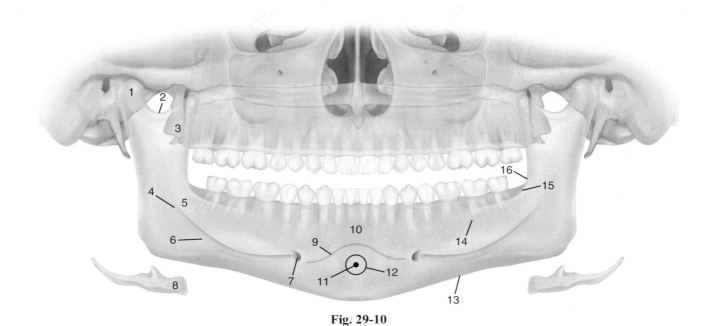

Fig. 29-10

Normal Anatomy of Mandible

Identify each structure labeled 1 to 16 in Fig. 29-10.

1. condyle
2. Sigmoid notch
3. coronoid process
4. mandibular foramen
5. lingula
6. mandibular canal
7. mental foramen
8. hyoid bone
9. mental ridge
10. mental fossa
11. lingual foramen
12. genial tubercle
13. inferior border of man.
14. mylohyoid ridge
15. internal oblique ridge
16. external oblique ridge

Module **6**   **Film Mounting, Normal Anatomy, and Interpretation Basics**

Kelsey Rubin

SHORT ANSWER

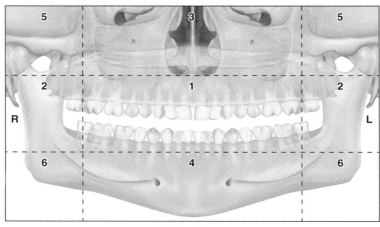

Fig. 29-11

Diagnostic Panoramic Image Features

For each of the six areas identified on Fig. 29-11, describe the features that should be visible to determine the **diagnostic quality** of the panoramic image. (See Box 22-1 in text.)

1. Area 1: Should include all teeth from molars to central incisors, stopping at hard + sot palte.

2. Area 2: Styloid process, hamulus, maxillary tuberosity lateral pterygoid plate, mastoid process, coronoid process, internal oblique ridge, external oblique ridge

3. Area 3: Orbit, nasal septum, incisive canal, anterior nasal spine, hard palate, infraorbital oramen, nasal cavity + conchae

4. Area 4: Mental fossa, mental ridge, lingual foramen, genial tubercles, inferior bordr of mandible, myolid ridge, man. canal, man. foramen, lingula

5. Area 5: Articular eminence, glenoid fossa, external auditory meatus, pterygomaxillary fissure, sigmoid notch, condyle, zygomatic arch, zygomatic process of maxilla

6. Area 6: Man. canal, man. foramen, lingula, hyoid bone,

For each panoramic image provided, complete a **Panoramic Image Interpretation Worksheet**. For each panoramic image, practice identifying normal anatomy.

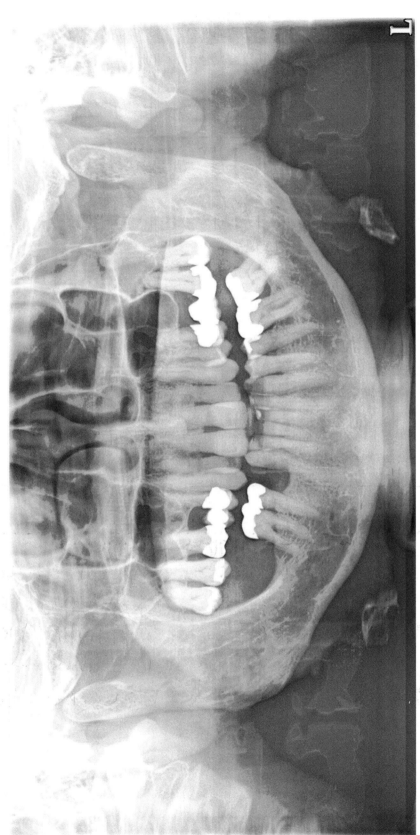

Fig. 29-12

PANORAMIC IMAGE
INTERPRETATION WORKSHEET

PAN NUMBER	29-12	
DIAGNOSTIC QUALITY	☐ no ☐ yes	
RETAKE NEEDED	☐ no ☐ yes	
ARTIFACTS	☐ no ☐ yes	*describe any artifacts here*

TEETH

BONE

TEETH			BONE		
IMPACTED TEETH *list numbers*	☐ no ☐ yes		**PERIAPICAL RADIOLUCENCY**	☐ no ☐ yes	*list location & estimate size*
NUMBER ANOMALIES *supernumerary or congenitally missing*	☐ no ☐ yes		**PERIAPICAL RADIOPACITY**	☐ no ☐ yes	*list location & estimate size*
CROWN ANOMALIES *size/shape defects*	☐ no ☐ yes		**NON–TOOTH-RELATED LESIONS**	☐ no ☐ yes	
CARIES, CALCULUS, DEFECTIVE RESTORATIONS	☐ no ☐ yes	*additional intraoral images are needed to evaluate*	**OTHER**	☐ no ☐ yes	

OTHER FINDINGS

MAXILLARY SINUS		**AREA BELOW OR LATERAL TO MANDIBLE**	
CONDYLE TMJ AREA		**MISCELLANEOUS**	
ADDITIONAL COMMENTS			

on diagram

- indicate the location of any periapical lesions
- indicate the location of any bone anomalies
- indicate with a ★ if any area requires further evaluation

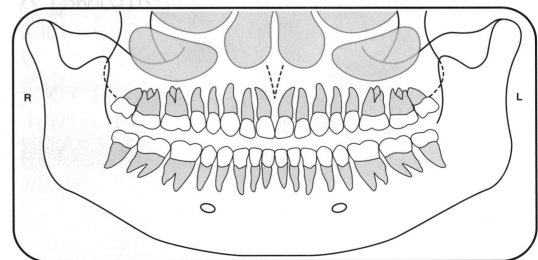

R   L

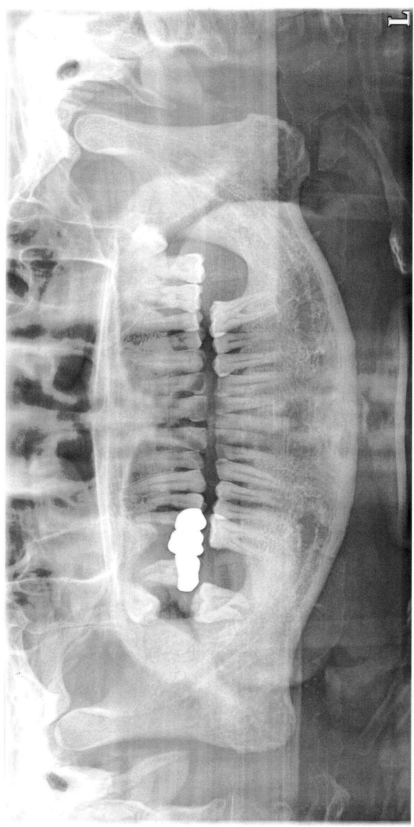

Fig. 29-16

PANORAMIC IMAGE
INTERPRETATION WORKSHEET

PAN NUMBER		
DIAGNOSTIC QUALITY	☐ no ☐ yes	
RETAKE NEEDED	☐ no ☐ yes	
ARTIFACTS	☐ no ☐ yes	*describe any artifacts here*

TEETH

BONE

TEETH			BONE		
IMPACTED TEETH *list numbers*	☐ no ☐ yes		**PERIAPICAL RADIOLUCENCY**	☐ no ☐ yes	*list location & estimate size*
NUMBER ANOMALIES *supernumerary or congenitally missing*	☐ no ☐ yes		**PERIAPICAL RADIOPACITY**	☐ no ☐ yes	*list location & estimate size*
CROWN ANOMALIES *size/shape defects*	☐ no ☐ yes		**NON–TOOTH-RELATED LESIONS**	☐ no ☐ yes	
CARIES, CALCULUS, DEFECTIVE RESTORATIONS	☐ no ☐ yes	*additional intraoral images are needed to evaluate*	**OTHER**	☐ no ☐ yes	

OTHER FINDINGS

MAXILLARY SINUS		**AREA BELOW OR LATERAL TO MANDIBLE**	
CONDYLE TMJ AREA		**MISCELLANEOUS**	
ADDITIONAL COMMENTS			

on diagram

- indicate the location of any periapical lesions
- indicate the location of any bone anomalies
- indicate with a ★ if any area requires further evaluation

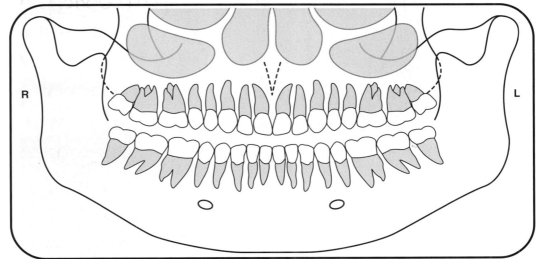

R   L

Module **6**   **Film Mounting, Normal Anatomy, and Interpretation Basics**

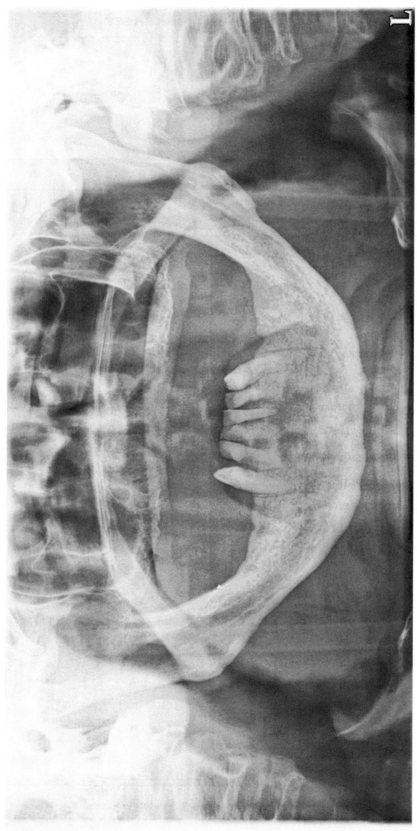

Fig. 29-17

PANORAMIC IMAGE
INTERPRETATION WORKSHEET

PAN NUMBER		
DIAGNOSTIC QUALITY	☐ no ☐ yes	
RETAKE NEEDED	☐ no ☐ yes	
ARTIFACTS	☐ no ☐ yes	*describe any artifacts here*

TEETH

			BONE		
IMPACTED TEETH *list numbers*	☐ no ☐ yes		**PERIAPICAL RADIOLUCENCY**	☐ no ☐ yes	*list location & estimate size*
NUMBER ANOMALIES *supernumerary or congenitally missing*	☐ no ☐ yes		**PERIAPICAL RADIOPACITY**	☐ no ☐ yes	*list location & estimate size*
CROWN ANOMALIES *size/shape defects*	☐ no ☐ yes		**NON–TOOTH-RELATED LESIONS**	☐ no ☐ yes	
CARIES, CALCULUS, DEFECTIVE RESTORATIONS	☐ no ☐ yes	*additional intraoral images are needed to evaluate*	**OTHER**	☐ no ☐ yes	

OTHER FINDINGS

MAXILLARY SINUS			**AREA BELOW OR LATERAL TO MANDIBLE**	
CONDYLE TMJ AREA			**MISCELLANEOUS**	
ADDITIONAL COMMENTS				

on diagram

- indicate the location of any periapical lesions
- indicate the location of any bone anomalies
- indicate with a ★ if any area requires further evaluation

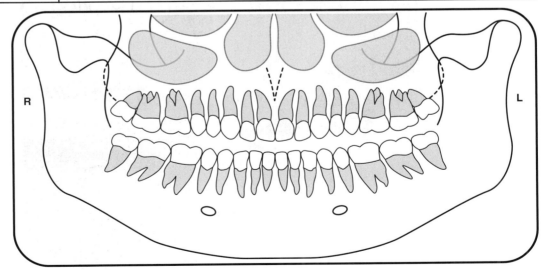

Module 6   **Film Mounting, Normal Anatomy, and Interpretation Basics**

WORKBOOK EXERCISES

Chapter 30   Introduction to Interpretation

ORDERING

Number the following in order of the **recommended viewing sequence** for interpretation of images.

1. _____ bite-wings—left

2. _____ bite-wings—right

3. _____ mandibular anterior periapicals

4. _____ mandibular posterior periapicals—left

5. _____ mandibular posterior periapicals—right

6. _____ maxillary anterior periapicals

7. _____ maxillary posterior periapicals—left

8. _____ maxillary posterior periapicals—right

TRUE OR FALSE

1. _____ The documentation of dental image interpretation is optional.

2. _____ The amount and scope of training in dental imaging determines whether the dental hygienist may establish a diagnosis.

3. _____ Interpretation of dental images is needed before treatment planning.

4. _____ Evaluation of the diagnostic quality of dental images is not part of interpretation documentation.

5. _____ A knowledge of normal anatomic structures is needed for image interpretation.

6. _____ A knowledge of common artifacts and errors is optional for image interpretation.

7. _____ It is recommended to obtain dental images at the end of the appointment.

8. _____ Dental images may be used for diagnostic, therapeutic, and educational purposes.

WORKBOOK EXERCISES

Chapter 31 Descriptive Terminology

SHORT ANSWER

For each image, describe the **appearance** and **location** of the lesion or condition.

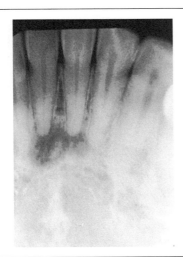	**1.**
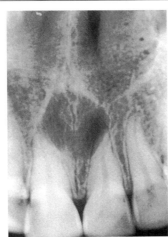	**2.**
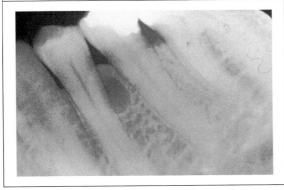	**3.**

Module **6** **Film Mounting, Normal Anatomy, and Interpretation Basics**

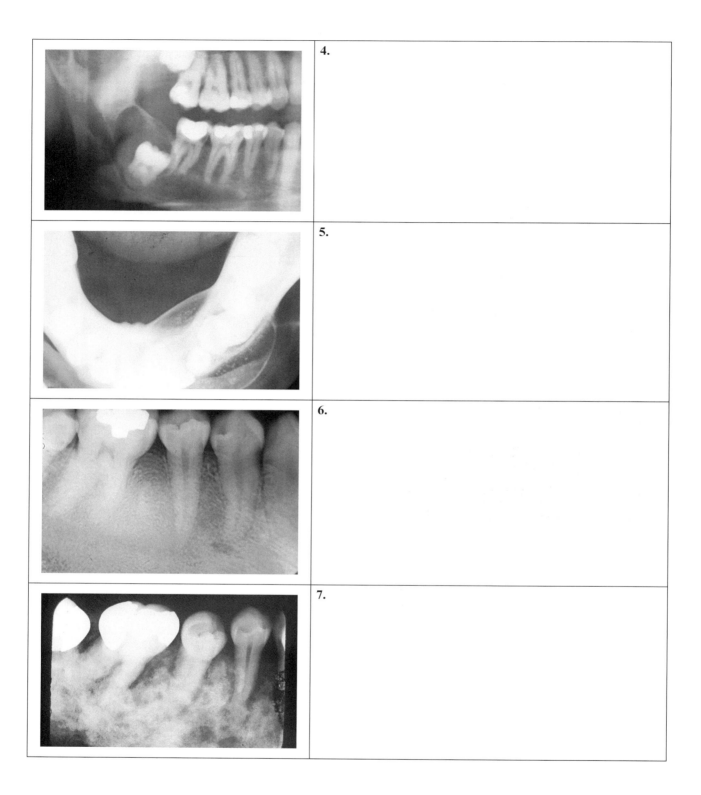

4.

5.

6.

7.

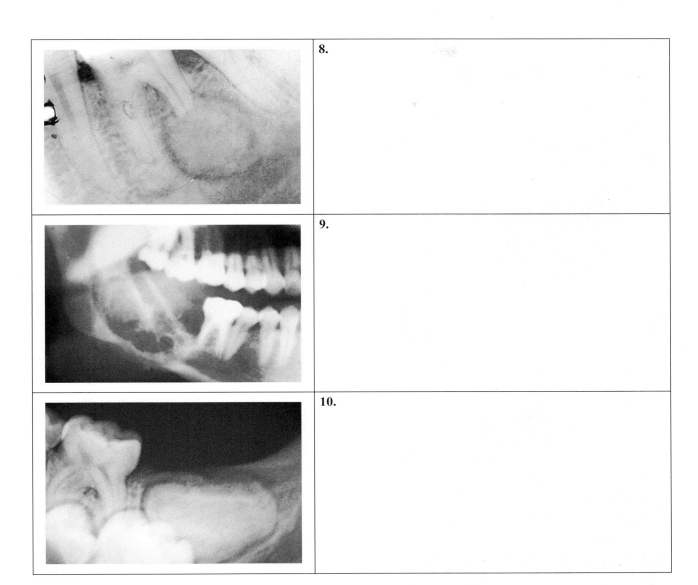

8.

9.

10.

Module **6** **Film Mounting, Normal Anatomy, and Interpretation Basics**

APPLICATION

Module 6 Film Mounting, Normal Anatomy, and Interpretation Basics

SELF-ASSESSMENT

Chapters 28 - 31

Based on the worksheets that you have just completed for Chapters 28 - 31, how prepared are you for the upcoming Module 6 assessments?

_____ very prepared, confident

_____ somewhat prepared, somewhat confident

_____ somewhat unprepared, lack confidence

_____ unprepared, no confidence

Based on your answer above, what is your plan for improvement? List the topics and concepts that you need to further review and study for assessments.

_____

_____

_____

_____

_____

_____

CRITICAL THINKING QUESTIONS

What does all the information in Chapters 28 to 31 mean to you in the practice setting? Use the questions below to help you apply the information that you have just learned. Work in pairs and practice answering these questions with your classmates. Share feedback concerning the content and delivery of information—is the information correct and understandable for the average patient? Are effective communication skills being used? The more you practice, the more comfortable you will be discussing these issues with your patients.

1. **A new assistant has started working in your office. It is your job to teach and instruct your new coworker on when, where, and why images are mounted and who mounts them. What important details will you share with the assistant?**

   • CHAPTER 28

2. **A student at the local university has come into your office for a career day. She is interested in becoming a part of the dental team and would like to see what each job entails and what it is like to be in the dental profession for a day. As you are explaining to her the daily routine of your office, she asks why you can interpret images but not diagnose. How can you answer the student correctly?**

   • CHAPTER 30

3. **After viewing a radiolucent periapical lesion on a dental image, what should the dental radiographer record in the patient's record?**

   • CHAPTER 31

4. **In dental imaging, a number of different terms can be used to describe the appearance, location, and size of a lesion. Why would you want to utilize descriptive terminology to discuss and describe what is seen on a dental image?**

   • CHAPTER 31

TO-DO CHECKLIST

Written Exercises

____ Complete all worksheets.

____ Complete self-assessment.

Active Learning Experiences

____ Complete all film/image mounting and normal anatomy exercises.

____ Practice mounting images using the Interactive Exercises on Evolve.

____ Practice mounting films, if available.

____ Work with an instructor to review normal anatomy on a human skull.

____ Review and answer the critical thinking questions.

____ Practice answering critical thinking questions with your classmates and provide feedback.

HOW TO MOUNT BITE-WINGS

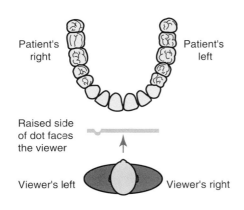

Patient's right   Patient's left

Raised side of dot faces the viewer

Viewer's left   Viewer's right

PREP
- Label mount
- Work on a light-colored surface
- Use a view box

ARRANGE
- **Dot:** place films with embossed **dot facing up**
- **Arrange:** arrange in **anatomic order** note **CURVE OF SPEE**

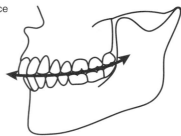

MOUNT
- Mount each BW film
- Start on left of mount
- Work from left to right
- For each film:
  – Slide film under middle two tabs (1)
  – Then slide under left tab (2)
  – Then click film into right tab (3)

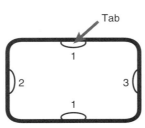

Tab

1

2   3

1

CHECK—CHECK—CHECK
- **Dots facing up?**
  All embossed dots are facing up
- **Correct location?**
  Each film is placed in correct mount location
- **Films secured?**
  Each film is secured with four plastic tabs

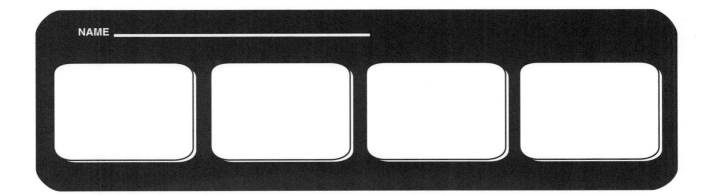

NAME

CURVE OF SPEE

- also known as the **occlusal plane**

- **convex** on the maxillary arch

- **concave** on the **mandibular** arch

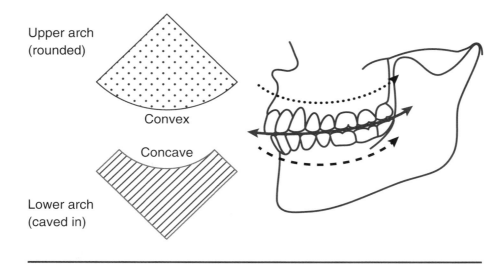

Upper arch (rounded)

Convex

Concave

Lower arch (caved in)

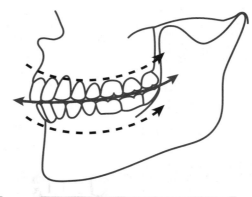

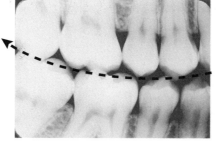

correct orientation

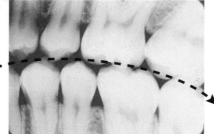

incorrect orientation

HOW TO MOUNT A COMPLETE SERIES

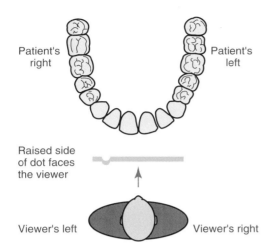

Patient's right

Patient's left

Raised side of dot faces the viewer

Viewer's left

Viewer's right

PREP
- Label mount
- Work on a light-colored surface
- Use a viewbox

ARRANGE
- **Dot:** place all films with embossed **dot facing up**
- **Sort: sort films** into BWs, anterior PAs and posterior PAs
- **Arrange:** arrange in **anatomic order**

MOUNT
- Mount each film
- Start on left of mount
- Work from L to R
- For each film:
  - Slide film under middle two tabs (1)
  - Then slide under left tab (2)
  - Then click film into right tab (3)

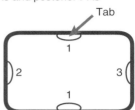

Tab

ORDER (see below)
- **First:** mount **Bite-wings** from L to R: 1, 2, 3, 4
- **Second:** mount MAXILLARY **Anterior PAs** from L to R: 5, 6, 7, 8
- **Next:** mount MANDIBULAR **Anterior PAs** from L to R: 9, 10, 11
- **Next:** mount MAXILLARY **Posterior PAs** from L to R: 12, 13, 14, 15
- **Last:** mount MANDIBULAR **Posterior PAs** from L to R: 16, 17, 18, 19

CHECK—CHECK—CHECK
- **Dots facing up?** all embossed dots are facing up
- **Correct location?** each film is placed in correct mount location
- **Films secured?** each film is secured with four plastic tabs

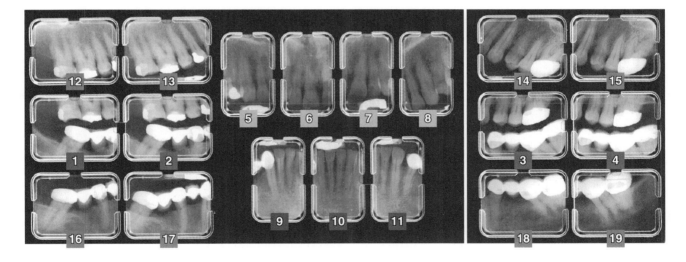

Module **6** **Film Mounting, Normal Anatomy, and Interpretation Basics**

INSTRUCTIONS

How to Prepare
- Review the learning objectives for Module 7 prior to lab.
- Review the critical thinking questions for Module 7 prior to lab.

What to Bring
- *Workbook and Laboratory Manual*—Module 7 materials
- pencil
- textbook (print or e-version)

Written Exercises
- Work together or individually to complete each interpretation exercise.
- When each interpretation is finished, use key to check answers; correct any wrong answers.
- Use your completed and corrected worksheets to study for assessments.

7 Interpretation Basics

LEARNING OBJECTIVES

The goal of Module 7 laboratory experiences is to provide students with a reinforcement of the fundamental understanding of image interpretation basics. Upon successful completion of Chapters 32 to 35 lectures and laboratory, the student will be able to complete interpretations on selected complete series of images as well as:

CHAPTER	LEARNING OBJECTIVES

CHAPTER 32   IDENTIFICATION OF RESTORATIONS, DENTAL MATERIALS, AND FOREIGN OBJECTS

Written Exercises	• Define key terms associated with identifying restorations, materials, and foreign objects on images. • On dental images, identify and describe the appearance of amalgam, gold, stainless steel, chrome, post and core, porcelain, porcelain-fused-to-metal, composite, and acrylic. • On dental images, identify and describe the appearance of base materials, metallic pins, gutta-percha, silver points, removable partial dentures, complete dentures, orthodontic bands, brackets and wires, fixed retainers, implants, suture wires, splints, and stabilizing arches. • On dental images, identify and describe the appearance of jewelry and eyeglasses.

CHAPTER 33   IDENTIFICATION OF DENTAL CARIES

Written Exercises	• Define the key terms associated with the interpretation of dental caries. • Describe dental caries. • Explain why caries appear radiolucent on a dental image. • Discuss interpretation tips for evaluating caries on a dental image. • Discuss the factors that may influence the image interpretation of dental caries.

CHAPTER 34   INTERPRETATION OF PERIODONTAL DISEASE

Written Exercises	• Define the key terms associated with interpreting periodontal disease. • Discuss the importance of the clinical examination and interpretation of dental images in the diagnosis of periodontal disease. • Describe the limitations of dental images in the detection of periodontal disease. • Describe the type of images that should be used to document periodontal disease and the preferred exposure technique.

CHAPTER 35   INTERPRETATION OF TRAUMA, PULPAL, AND PERIAPICAL LESIONS

Written Exercises	• Define the key terms associated with the interpretation of trauma, pulpal lesions, and periapical lesions viewed on a dental image. • Describe and identify the appearance of crown, root, and jaw fractures viewed on a dental image. • Describe and identify the appearance of an avulsion viewed on a dental image. • Describe and identify the appearance of internal and external resorption viewed on a dental image. • Describe and identify the appearance of a periapical granuloma, cyst, and abscess viewed on a dental image. • Describe and identify the appearance of condensing osteitis, sclerotic bone, and hypercementosis viewed on a dental image.

WORKBOOK EXERCISES

Chapters 32-35   Interpretation Basics

DENTAL IMAGES AND INTERPRETATION REVIEW

Why Are Dental Images Important?

- Dental images are an essential part of the patient record.

- Dental images play a critical role in diagnosis and patient care.

- Dental images document a patient's condition at a specific point in time.

- Dental images allow for the gathering of information about diseases, lesions, and conditions of teeth and jaws, which cannot be identified clinically.

What Is Image Interpretation?

- It is the explanation or description of what is viewed on a dental image.

- It is *not* a diagnosis; it is only a part of the information that is required to establish a diagnosis.

- Interpretation refers to a description of image findings.

- Diagnosis refers to the identification of disease by examination or analysis.

- A diagnosis must be established by a dentist.

- In order to establish a diagnosis, a thorough review of the medical history, dental history, clinical examination, image interpretation, and clinical or laboratory tests is needed.

What Training Is Needed for Interpretation?

- Students must be confident in the identification of normal anatomy, restorations, dental materials, foreign objects, dental caries, periodontal disease, traumatic injuries, pulpal changes, periapical lesions, lesions of bone, and bone anomalies.

- Training includes lectures on the topic of image interpretation and ongoing experiences in the clinical setting.

What Is Documented?

All dental images must be reviewed and interpreted. The interpretation, or description of image findings, must be documented in the patient record and include the following:

- number and type of images

- date of exposure

- evaluation of diagnostic quality

- list of limiting factors, retakes, or additional images needed

- description of teeth—indicate impactions, number anomalies, crown anomalies, defective restorations, caries, calculus, pulpal changes, root abnormalities, and other miscellaneous features

- description of bone and supporting structures of the teeth—indicate periapical radiolucencies and radiopacities, bone loss, changes in crestal lamina dura and radicular lamina dura, changes in periodontal ligament space, any furcation involvement, interdental trabecular pattern of bone, any lesions of bone or bone anomalies

- description of artifacts

- indication of any areas that require additional imaging or clinical evaluation and confirmation

283

DENTAL IMAGE INTERPRETATION FORM

What Is the Dental Image Interpretation Form?

In an effort to provide consistent interpretation experiences for students, the Dental Image Interpretation Form was created to document image findings. It is important to note that the purpose of the worksheet is to identify image findings only and additional clinical information is required to establish a definitive diagnosis.

Why Use the Dental Image Interpretation Form?

In the absence of a worksheet, a detailed narrative description of image findings is needed in the patient record. To write a narrative description that includes all the information that needs to be documented is time consuming to prepare and subject to a variety of inconsistencies.

An example of such a narrative description appears below:

7-1-2016

12 periapicals, 2 bite-wings, and panoramic image reviewed with instructor. Images are diagnostic. No additional intraoral images or retakes needed. Limiting factors included a gag reflex stimulated by posterior periapical placements. Impacted teeth #1, 16, 17, 32 noted.

Multiple broken teeth, defective restorations, caries, and previous RCT noted. Root tips present in posterior left maxilla. Extra root noted on tooth #20. Periapical radiolucency present on tooth #6 (~5 mm in diameter) and tooth #23 (~4 mm in diameter). Well-defined radiopacity (~4 mm in diameter) suggestive of sclerotic bone noted in right posterior mandible.

Generalized moderate-to-severe bone loss present in maxilla and mandible; crestal lamina dura is fuzzy and indistinct. Multiple furcation involvements noted. See restorative and periodontal charting for specific details. On panoramic image, ghost images caused by small earrings noted on right and left sides.

How Does the Dental Image Interpretation Form Assist the Student in Learning?

As an alternative to a narrative description, the Dental Image Interpretation Form has been designed to assist the student in learning interpretation skills by providing the following:

- an organized format to gather essential information that is needed before diagnosis and treatment planning

- a defined process to follow that serves as a roadmap for consistency

- a step-by-step list of what to examine on dental images

- a list of findings to verify clinically

- a format for self-evaluation of interpretation skills

DENTAL IMAGE
INTERPRETATION FORM

IMAGES	# OF IMAGES _____BW _____PA _____PAN		
DIAGNOSTIC QUALITY	☐ no ☐ yes	**ADDITIONAL IMAGES NEEDED**	☐ no ☐ yes *list on reverse side*
RETAKES	☐ no ☐ yes *list on reverse side*	**LIMITING FACTORS**	☐ no ☐ yes *list on reverse side*

TEETH

IMPACTED TEETH	☐ no ☐ n/a*	☐ yes	**PULP CAVITY FEATURES**	☐ normal ☐ pulp stones
				☐ sclerotic ☐ resorption
NUMBER ANOMALIES supernumerary teeth / congenitally missing teeth	☐ no ☐ n/a*	☐ yes	☐ n/a*	☐ obliterated ☐ previous RCT
				☐ other
CROWN ANOMALIES size / shape defects	☐ no ☐ n/a*	☐ yes	**ROOT FEATURES**	☐ normal ☐ short or long
				☐ root tips ☐ extra roots
DEFECTIVE RESTORATIONS overhang / open contacts	☐ no ☐ n/a*	☐ yes *list on reverse side*	☐ n/a*	☐ root fracture ☐ dilacerations
				☐ resorption ☐ hypercementosis
CARIES suspicious areas to be evaluated clinically	☐ no ☐ n/a*	☐ yes *list on reverse side*	**MISCELLANEOUS FEATURES**	☐ none ☐ attrition
				☐ implants ☐ abrasion
CALCULUS	☐ no ☐ n/a*	☐ yes	☐ n/a*	☐ other ☐ trauma

BONE

PERIAPICAL AREA radiolucency	☐ no ☐ n/a*	☐ yes *list on reverse*	**LAMINA DURA** crestal ☐ n/a*	☐ intact ☐ fuzzy, indistinct
				☐ notched
PERIAPICAL AREA radiopacity	☐ no ☐ n/a*	☐ yes *list on reverse*	**LAMINA DURA** radicular ☐ n/a*	☐ normal ☐ thickened
				☐ absent
BONE LOSS percent & pattern	☐ no bone loss ☐ n/a*		**PDL SPACE** ☐ n/a*	☐ normal ☐ widened
				☐ obliterated
	☐ ≤20% *slight* L *or* G		**FURCATION INVOLVEMENT** ☐ n/a*	☐ none ☐ wide pdl in furcation
	☐ 21- 49% *moderate* L *or* G			☐ ≤3 furcations
	☐ ≥50% *severe* L *or* G			☐ ≥4 furcations
	☐ horizontal ☐ vertical		**INTERDENTAL TRABECULATIONS** ☐ n/a*	☐ normal ☐ ↑ bone density
				☐ ↓ bone density
BONE ANOMALIES non–tooth-related lesions	☐ no ☐ n/a*	☐ yes *list on reverse side*	**OTHER** ☐ n/a*	☐ document on reverse	***n/a** *cannot be determined from images reviewed; additional images needed*

DENTAL IMAGE INTERPRETATION FORM

IMAGES	# OF IMAGES 4 BW 14 PA ☒ PAN		SERIES 1	
DIAGNOSTIC QUALITY	☐ no	☒ yes	**ADDITIONAL IMAGES NEEDED** ☐ no ☒ yes	*list on reverse side*
RETAKES	☐ no	☒ yes *list on reverse side*	**LIMITING FACTORS** ☐ no ☐ yes	*list on reverse side*

TEETH

IMPACTED TEETH	☒ no ☐ n/a*	☐ yes	**PULP CAVITY FEATURES** ☐ n/a*	☐ normal ☐ sclerotic ☐ obliterated ☐ other	☐ pulp stones ☐ resorption ☐ previous RCT
NUMBER ANOMALIES supernumerary teeth / congenitally missing teeth	☒ no ☐ n/a*	☐ yes			
CROWN ANOMALIES size / shape defects	☒ no ☐ n/a*	☐ yes	**ROOT FEATURES** ☐ n/a*	☐ normal ☐ root tips ☐ root fracture ☐ resorption	☐ short or long ☐ extra roots ☐ dilacerations ☐ hypercementosis
DEFECTIVE RESTORATIONS overhang / open contacts	☐ no ☐ n/a*	☒ yes *list on reverse side*			
CARIES suspicious areas to be evaluated clinically	☐ no ☐ n/a*	☐ yes *list on reverse side*	**MISCELLANEOUS FEATURES** ☐ n/a*	☐ none ☐ implants ☐ other	☐ attrition ☐ abrasion ☐ trauma
CALCULUS	☐ no ☐ n/a*	☐ yes			

BONE

PERIAPICAL AREA radiolucency	☐ no ☐ n/a*	☐ yes *list on reverse*	**LAMINA DURA** crestal ☐ n/a*	☐ intact	☐ fuzzy, indistinct ☐ notched
PERIAPICAL AREA radiopacity	☐ no ☐ n/a*	☐ yes *list on reverse*	**LAMINA DURA** radicular ☐ n/a*	☒ normal	☐ thickened ☐ absent
BONE LOSS percent & pattern	☐ no bone loss ☐ n/a*		**PDL SPACE** ☐ n/a*	☐ normal	☐ widened ☐ obliterated
	☐ ≤20% *slight* L or G ☐ 21-49% *moderate* L or G ☐ ≥50% *severe* L or G		**FURCATION INVOLVEMENT** ☐ n/a*	☐ none	☐ wide pdl in furcation ☐ ≤3 furcations ☐ ≥4 furcations
	☐ horizontal ☐ vertical		**INTERDENTAL TRABECULATIONS** ☐ n/a*	☐ normal	☐ ↑ bone density ☐ ↓ bone density
BONE ANOMALIES non–tooth-related lesions	☐ no ☐ n/a*	☐ yes *list on reverse side*	**OTHER** ☐ n/a*	☐ document on reverse	***n/a** *cannot be determined from images reviewed; additional images needed*

ADDITIONAL NOTES

TEETH

IMPACTED TEETH			**PULP CAVITY FEATURES**		
NUMBER ANOMALIES supernumerary teeth / congenitally missing teeth					
CROWN ANOMALIES size / shape defects			**ROOT FEATURES**		
DEFECTIVE RESTORATIONS overhang / open contacts					

CARIES suspicious areas to be evaluated clinically tooth numbers listed indicate surface (mesial) M (distal) D (occlusal) O	1		17		**MISCELLANEOUS FEATURES**
	2		18		
	3		19		
	4		20		
	5		21		
	6		22		
	7		23		
	8		24		
	9		25		
	10		26		
	11		27		
	12		28		
	13		29		
	14		30		
	15		31		
	16		32		

BONE

PERIAPICAL AREA radiolucency		**LAMINA DURA** crestal	
PERIAPICAL AREA radiopacity		**LAMINA DURA** radicular	
BONE LOSS percent & pattern		**PDL SPACE**	
		FURCATION INVOLVEMENT	
		INTERDENTAL TRABECULATIONS	
BONE ANOMALIES non–tooth-related lesions		**OTHER**	

IMAGES NEEDED

list additional images needed	

Series 2

Complete a dental image interpretation form for the series in Fig. 32-10.

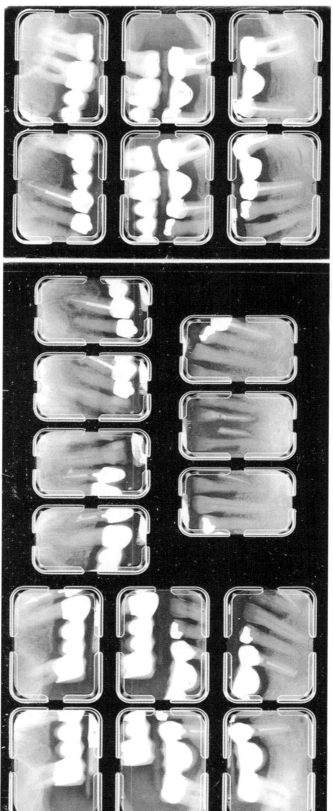

Fig. 32-10

Module **7** **Interpretation Basics**

DENTAL IMAGE
INTERPRETATION FORM

IMAGES	# OF IMAGES ____BW ____PA ____PAN		SERIES 2		
DIAGNOSTIC QUALITY	☐ no	☐ yes	**ADDITIONAL IMAGES NEEDED**	☐ no ☐ yes	*list on reverse side*
RETAKES	☐ no	☐ yes *list on reverse side*	**LIMITING FACTORS**	☐ no ☐ yes	*list on reverse side*

TEETH

IMPACTED TEETH	☐ no ☐ n/a*	☐ yes	**PULP CAVITY FEATURES** ☐ n/a*	☐ normal ☐ sclerotic ☐ obliterated ☐ other	☐ pulp stones ☐ resorption ☐ previous RCT
NUMBER ANOMALIES supernumerary teeth / congenitally missing teeth	☐ no ☐ n/a*	☐ yes			
CROWN ANOMALIES size / shape defects	☐ no ☐ n/a*	☐ yes	**ROOT FEATURES** ☐ n/a*	☐ normal ☐ root tips ☐ root fracture ☐ resorption	☐ short or long ☐ extra roots ☐ dilacerations ☐ hypercementosis
DEFECTIVE RESTORATIONS overhang / open contacts	☐ no ☐ n/a*	☐ yes *list on reverse side*			
CARIES suspicious areas to be evaluated clinically	☐ no ☐ n/a*	☐ yes *list on reverse side*	**MISCELLANEOUS FEATURES** ☐ n/a*	☐ none ☐ implants ☐ other	☐ attrition ☐ abrasion ☐ trauma
CALCULUS	☐ no ☐ n/a*	☐ yes			

BONE

PERIAPICAL AREA radiolucency	☐ no ☐ n/a*	☐ yes *list on reverse*	**LAMINA DURA** crestal ☐ n/a*	☐ intact	☐ fuzzy, indistinct ☐ notched
PERIAPICAL AREA radiopacity	☐ no ☐ n/a*	☐ yes *list on reverse*	**LAMINA DURA** radicular ☐ n/a*	☐ normal	☐ thickened ☐ absent
BONE LOSS percent & pattern	☐ no bone loss ☐ n/a*		**PDL SPACE** ☐ n/a*	☐ normal	☐ widened ☐ obliterated
	☐ ≤20% *slight* *L or G* ☐ 21-49% *moderate* *L or G* ☐ ≥50% *severe* *L or G*		**FURCATION INVOLVEMENT** ☐ n/a*	☐ none	☐ wide pdl in furcation ☐ ≤3 furcations ☐ ≥4 furcations
	☐ horizontal ☐ vertical		**INTERDENTAL TRABECULATIONS** ☐ n/a*	☐ normal	☐ ↑ bone density ☐ ↓ bone density
BONE ANOMALIES non–tooth-related lesions	☐ no ☐ n/a*	☐ yes *list on reverse side*	**OTHER** ☐ n/a*	☐ document on reverse	***n/a** *cannot be determined from images reviewed; additional images needed*

ADDITIONAL NOTES

TEETH

IMPACTED TEETH			**PULP CAVITY FEATURES**	
NUMBER ANOMALIES supernumerary teeth / congenitally missing teeth				
CROWN ANOMALIES size / shape defects			**ROOT FEATURES**	
DEFECTIVE RESTORATIONS overhang / open contacts				

CARIES suspicious areas to be evaluated clinically tooth numbers listed indicate surface (mesial) M (distal) D (occlusal) O	1		17	
	2		18	
	3		19	
	4		20	
	5		21	
	6		22	
	7		23	
	8		24	
	9		25	
	10		26	
	11		27	
	12		28	
	13		29	
	14		30	
	15		31	
	16		32	

MISCELLANEOUS FEATURES

BONE

PERIAPICAL AREA radiolucency		**LAMINA DURA** crestal	
PERIAPICAL AREA radiopacity		**LAMINA DURA** radicular	
BONE LOSS percent & pattern		**PDL SPACE**	
		FURCATION INVOLVEMENT	
		INTERDENTAL TRABECULATIONS	
BONE ANOMALIES non–tooth-related lesions		**OTHER**	

IMAGES NEEDED

list additional images needed	

Series 3

Complete a dental image interpretation form for the series in Fig. 32-11.

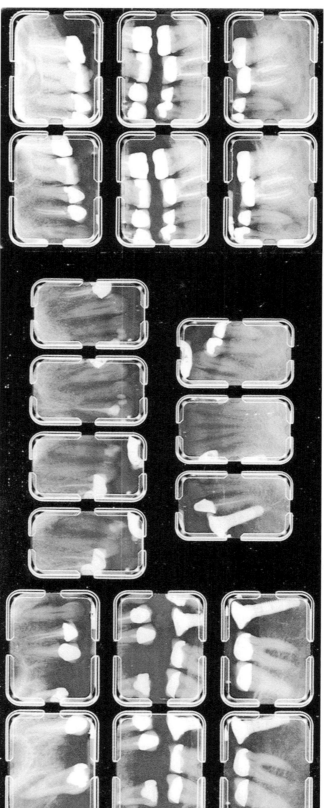

Fig. 32-11

DENTAL IMAGE
INTERPRETATION FORM

IMAGES	# OF IMAGES ____BW ____PA ____PAN		SERIES 3		
DIAGNOSTIC QUALITY	☐ no	☐ yes	**ADDITIONAL IMAGES NEEDED**	☐ no ☐ yes	*list on reverse side*
RETAKES	☐ no	☐ yes *list on reverse side*	**LIMITING FACTORS**	☐ no ☐ yes	*list on reverse side*

TEETH

IMPACTED TEETH	☐ no ☐ n/a*	☐ yes	**PULP CAVITY FEATURES** ☐ n/a*	☐ normal ☐ sclerotic ☐ obliterated ☐ other	☐ pulp stones ☐ resorption ☐ previous RCT
NUMBER ANOMALIES supernumerary teeth / congenitally missing teeth	☐ no ☐ n/a*	☐ yes			
CROWN ANOMALIES size / shape defects	☐ no ☐ n/a*	☐ yes	**ROOT FEATURES** ☐ n/a*	☐ normal ☐ root tips ☐ root fracture ☐ resorption	☐ short or long ☐ extra roots ☐ dilacerations ☐ hypercementosis
DEFECTIVE RESTORATIONS overhang / open contacts	☐ no ☐ n/a*	☐ yes *list on reverse side*			
CARIES suspicious areas to be evaluated clinically	☐ no ☐ n/a*	☐ yes *list on reverse side*	**MISCELLANEOUS FEATURES** ☐ n/a*	☐ none ☐ implants ☐ other	☐ attrition ☐ abrasion ☐ trauma
CALCULUS	☐ no ☐ n/a*	☐ yes			

BONE

PERIAPICAL AREA radiolucency	☐ no ☐ n/a*	☐ yes *list on reverse*	**LAMINA DURA** crestal ☐ n/a*	☐ intact	☐ fuzzy, indistinct ☐ notched
PERIAPICAL AREA radiopacity	☐ no ☐ n/a*	☐ yes *list on reverse*	**LAMINA DURA** radicular ☐ n/a*	☐ normal	☐ thickened ☐ absent
BONE LOSS percent & pattern	☐ no bone loss ☐ n/a*		**PDL SPACE** ☐ n/a*	☐ normal	☐ widened ☐ obliterated
	☐ ≤20% *slight* L or G ☐ 21- 49% *moderate* L or G ☐ ≥50% *severe* L or G		**FURCATION INVOLVEMENT** ☐ n/a*	☐ none	☐ wide pdl in furcation ☐ ≤3 furcations ☐ ≥4 furcations
	☐ horizontal ☐ vertical		**INTERDENTAL TRABECULATIONS** ☐ n/a*	☐ normal	☐ ↑ bone density ☐ ↓ bone density
BONE ANOMALIES non–tooth-related lesions	☐ no ☐ n/a*	☐ yes *list on reverse side*	**OTHER** ☐ n/a*	☐ document on reverse	***n/a** *cannot be determined from images reviewed; additional images needed*

ADDITIONAL NOTES

TEETH

IMPACTED TEETH		PULP CAVITY FEATURES	
NUMBER ANOMALIES supernumerary teeth / congenitally missing teeth			
CROWN ANOMALIES size / shape defects		ROOT FEATURES	
DEFECTIVE RESTORATIONS overhang / open contacts			

CARIES suspicious areas to be evaluated clinically tooth numbers listed indicate surface (mesial) M (distal) D (occlusal) O	1		17		MISCELLANEOUS FEATURES	
	2		18			
	3		19			
	4		20			
	5		21			
	6		22			
	7		23			
	8		24			
	9		25			
	10		26			
	11		27			
	12		28			
	13		29			
	14		30			
	15		31			
	16		32			

BONE

PERIAPICAL AREA radiolucency		LAMINA DURA crestal	
PERIAPICAL AREA radiopacity		LAMINA DURA radicular	
BONE LOSS percent & pattern		PDL SPACE	
		FURCATION INVOLVEMENT	
		INTERDENTAL TRABECULATIONS	
BONE ANOMALIES non–tooth-related lesions		OTHER	

IMAGES NEEDED

list additional images needed	

Series 4

Complete a dental image interpretation form for the series in Fig. 32-12.

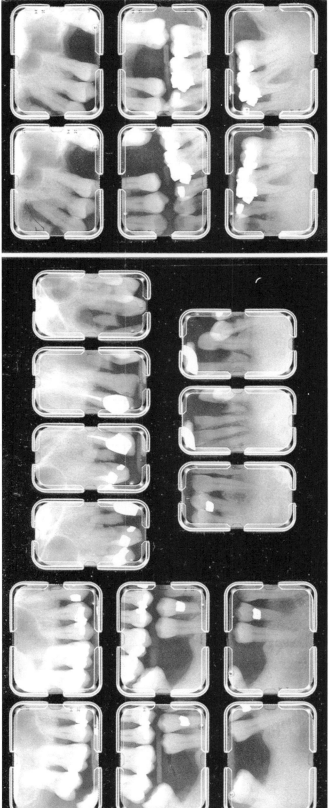

Fig. 32-12

DENTAL IMAGE
INTERPRETATION FORM

IMAGES	# OF IMAGES _____BW _____PA _____PAN		SERIES 4		
DIAGNOSTIC QUALITY	☐ no ☐ yes	**ADDITIONAL IMAGES NEEDED**	☐ no ☐ yes		*list on reverse side*
RETAKES	☐ no ☐ yes *list on reverse side*	**LIMITING FACTORS**	☐ no ☐ yes		*list on reverse side*

TEETH

IMPACTED TEETH	☐ no ☐ n/a*	☐ yes	**PULP CAVITY FEATURES** ☐ n/a*	☐ normal ☐ sclerotic ☐ obliterated ☐ other	☐ pulp stones ☐ resorption ☐ previous RCT
NUMBER ANOMALIES supernumerary teeth / congenitally missing teeth	☐ no ☐ n/a*	☐ yes			
CROWN ANOMALIES size / shape defects	☐ no ☐ n/a*	☐ yes	**ROOT FEATURES** ☐ n/a*	☐ normal ☐ root tips ☐ root fracture ☐ resorption	☐ short or long ☐ extra roots ☐ dilacerations ☐ hypercementosis
DEFECTIVE RESTORATIONS overhang / open contacts	☐ no ☐ n/a*	☐ yes *list on reverse side*			
CARIES suspicious areas to be evaluated clinically	☐ no ☐ n/a*	☐ yes *list on reverse side*	**MISCELLANEOUS FEATURES** ☐ n/a*	☐ none ☐ implants ☐ other	☐ attrition ☐ abrasion ☐ trauma
CALCULUS	☐ no ☐ n/a*	☐ yes			

BONE

PERIAPICAL AREA radiolucency	☐ no ☐ n/a*	☐ yes *list on reverse*	**LAMINA DURA** crestal ☐ n/a*	☐ intact	☐ fuzzy, indistinct ☐ notched
PERIAPICAL AREA radiopacity	☐ no ☐ n/a*	☐ yes *list on reverse*	**LAMINA DURA** radicular ☐ n/a*	☐ normal	☐ thickened ☐ absent
BONE LOSS percent & pattern		☐ no bone loss ☐ n/a*	**PDL SPACE** ☐ n/a*	☐ normal	☐ widened ☐ obliterated
		☐ ≤20% *slight* L or G ☐ 21- 49% *moderate* L or G ☐ ≥50% *severe* L or G	**FURCATION INVOLVEMENT** ☐ n/a*	☐ none	☐ wide pdl in furcation ☐ ≤3 furcations ☐ ≥4 furcations
		☐ horizontal ☐ vertical	**INTERDENTAL TRABECULATIONS** ☐ n/a*	☐ normal	☐ ↑ bone density ☐ ↓ bone density
BONE ANOMALIES non–tooth-related lesions	☐ no ☐ n/a*	☐ yes *list on reverse side*	**OTHER** ☐ n/a*	☐ document on reverse	*n/a cannot be determined from images reviewed; additional images needed

ADDITIONAL NOTES

TEETH

IMPACTED TEETH		**PULP CAVITY FEATURES**
NUMBER ANOMALIES supernumerary teeth / congenitally missing teeth		
CROWN ANOMALIES size / shape defects		**ROOT FEATURES**
DEFECTIVE RESTORATIONS overhang / open contacts		

CARIES suspicious areas to be evaluated clinically tooth numbers listed indicate surface (mesial) M (distal) D (occlusal) O	1		17		MISCELLANEOUS FEATURES
	2		18		
	3		19		
	4		20		
	5		21		
	6		22		
	7		23		
	8		24		
	9		25		
	10		26		
	11		27		
	12		28		
	13		29		
	14		30		
	15		31		
	16		32		

BONE

PERIAPICAL AREA radiolucency		**LAMINA DURA** crestal
PERIAPICAL AREA radiopacity		**LAMINA DURA** radicular
BONE LOSS percent & pattern		**PDL SPACE**
		FURCATION INVOLVEMENT
		INTERDENTAL TRABECULATIONS
BONE ANOMALIES non–tooth-related lesions		**OTHER**

IMAGES NEEDED

list additional images needed	

Complete a dental image interpretation form for the bite-wings in Fig. 32-13.

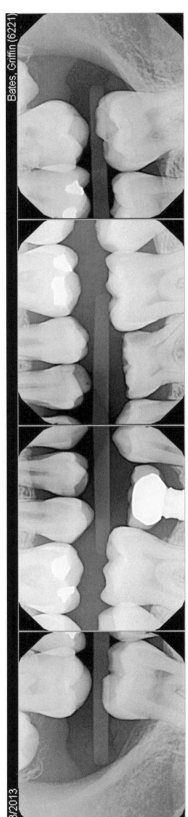

Fig. 32-13

306

DENTAL IMAGE
INTERPRETATION FORM

IMAGES	# OF IMAGES ____BW ____PA ____PAN	SERIES 5	
DIAGNOSTIC QUALITY	☐ no ☐ yes	**ADDITIONAL IMAGES NEEDED**	☐ no ☐ yes *list on reverse side*
RETAKES	☐ no ☐ yes *list on reverse side*	**LIMITING FACTORS**	☐ no ☐ yes *list on reverse side*

TEETH

IMPACTED TEETH	☐ no ☐ n/a* ☐ yes	**PULP CAVITY FEATURES** ☐ n/a*	☐ normal ☐ pulp stones ☐ sclerotic ☐ resorption ☐ obliterated ☐ previous RCT ☐ other
NUMBER ANOMALIES supernumerary teeth / congenitally missing teeth	☐ no ☐ n/a* ☐ yes		
CROWN ANOMALIES size / shape defects	☐ no ☐ n/a* ☐ yes	**ROOT FEATURES** ☐ n/a*	☐ normal ☐ short or long ☐ root tips ☐ extra roots ☐ root fracture ☐ dilacerations ☐ resorption ☐ hypercementosis
DEFECTIVE RESTORATIONS overhang / open contacts	☐ no ☐ n/a* ☐ yes *list on reverse side*		
CARIES suspicious areas to be evaluated clinically	☐ no ☐ n/a* ☐ yes *list on reverse side*	**MISCELLANEOUS FEATURES** ☐ n/a*	☐ none ☐ attrition ☐ implants ☐ abrasion ☐ other ☐ trauma
CALCULUS	☐ no ☐ n/a* ☐ yes		

BONE

PERIAPICAL AREA radiolucency	☐ no ☐ n/a* ☐ yes *list on reverse*	**LAMINA DURA** crestal ☐ n/a*	☐ intact ☐ fuzzy, indistinct ☐ notched
PERIAPICAL AREA radiopacity	☐ no ☐ n/a* ☐ yes *list on reverse*	**LAMINA DURA** radicular ☐ n/a*	☐ normal ☐ thickened ☐ absent
BONE LOSS percent & pattern	☐ no bone loss ☐ n/a*	**PDL SPACE** ☐ n/a*	☐ normal ☐ widened ☐ obliterated
	☐ ≤20% *slight* L or G ☐ 21-49% *moderate* L or G ☐ ≥50% *severe* L or G	**FURCATION INVOLVEMENT** ☐ n/a*	☐ none ☐ wide pdl in furcation ☐ ≤3 furcations ☐ ≥4 furcations
	☐ horizontal ☐ vertical	**INTERDENTAL TRABECULATIONS** ☐ n/a*	☐ normal ☐ ↑ bone density ☐ ↓ bone density
BONE ANOMALIES non–tooth-related lesions	☐ no ☐ n/a* ☐ yes *list on reverse side*	**OTHER** ☐ n/a*	☐ document on reverse ***n/a** *cannot be determined from images reviewed; additional images needed*

ADDITIONAL NOTES

TEETH

					PULP CAVITY FEATURES	
IMPACTED TEETH					**PULP CAVITY FEATURES**	
NUMBER ANOMALIES supernumerary teeth / congenitally missing teeth						
CROWN ANOMALIES size / shape defects					**ROOT FEATURES**	
DEFECTIVE RESTORATIONS overhang / open contacts						

CARIES suspicious areas to be evaluated clinically tooth numbers listed indicate surface (mesial) M (distal) D (occlusal) O	1		17		**MISCELLANEOUS FEATURES**	
	2		18			
	3		19			
	4		20			
	5		21			
	6		22			
	7		23			
	8		24			
	9		25			
	10		26			
	11		27			
	12		28			
	13		29			
	14		30			
	15		31			
	16		32			

BONE

PERIAPICAL AREA radiolucency		**LAMINA DURA** crestal	
PERIAPICAL AREA radiopacity		**LAMINA DURA** radicular	
BONE LOSS percent & pattern		**PDL SPACE**	
		FURCATION INVOLVEMENT	
		INTERDENTAL TRABECULATIONS	
BONE ANOMALIES non–tooth-related lesions		**OTHER**	

IMAGES NEEDED

list additional images needed	

Series 6

Complete a dental image interpretation form for the series in Fig. 32-14.

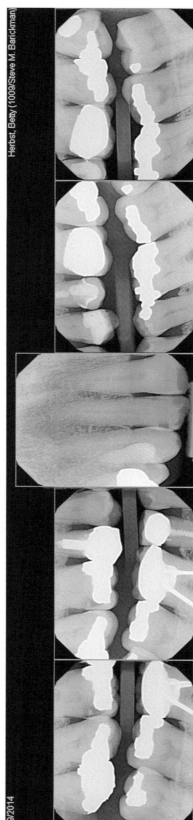

Fig. 32-14

DENTAL IMAGE
INTERPRETATION FORM

IMAGES	# OF IMAGES _____ BW _____ PA _____ PAN		SERIES 6		
DIAGNOSTIC QUALITY	☐ no	☐ yes	**ADDITIONAL IMAGES NEEDED**	☐ no ☐ yes	*list on reverse side*
RETAKES	☐ no	☐ yes *list on reverse side*	**LIMITING FACTORS**	☐ no ☐ yes	*list on reverse side*

TEETH

IMPACTED TEETH	☐ no ☐ n/a*	☐ yes	**PULP CAVITY FEATURES** ☐ n/a*	☐ normal ☐ sclerotic ☐ obliterated ☐ other	☐ pulp stones ☐ resorption ☐ previous RCT
NUMBER ANOMALIES supernumerary teeth / congenitally missing teeth	☐ no ☐ n/a*	☐ yes			
CROWN ANOMALIES size / shape defects	☐ no ☐ n/a*	☐ yes	**ROOT FEATURES** ☐ n/a*	☐ normal ☐ root tips ☐ root fracture ☐ resorption	☐ short or long ☐ extra roots ☐ dilacerations ☐ hypercementosis
DEFECTIVE RESTORATIONS overhang / open contacts	☐ no ☐ n/a*	☐ yes *list on reverse side*			
CARIES suspicious areas to be evaluated clinically	☐ no ☐ n/a*	☐ yes *list on reverse side*	**MISCELLANEOUS FEATURES** ☐ n/a*	☐ none ☐ implants ☐ other	☐ attrition ☐ abrasion ☐ trauma
CALCULUS	☐ no ☐ n/a*	☐ yes			

BONE

PERIAPICAL AREA radiolucency	☐ no ☐ n/a*	☐ yes *list on reverse*	**LAMINA DURA** crestal ☐ n/a*	☐ intact	☐ fuzzy, indistinct ☐ notched
PERIAPICAL AREA radiopacity	☐ no ☐ n/a*	☐ yes *list on reverse*	**LAMINA DURA** radicular ☐ n/a*	☐ normal	☐ thickened ☐ absent
BONE LOSS percent & pattern	☐ no bone loss ☐ n/a*	☐ ≤20% *slight* L or G ☐ 21- 49% *moderate* L or G ☐ ≥50% *severe* L or G	**PDL SPACE** ☐ n/a*	☐ normal	☐ widened ☐ obliterated
			FURCATION INVOLVEMENT ☐ n/a*	☐ none	☐ wide pdl in furcation ☐ ≤3 furcations ☐ ≥4 furcations
	☐ horizontal ☐ vertical		**INTERDENTAL TRABECULATIONS** ☐ n/a*	☐ normal	☐ ↑ bone density ☐ ↓ bone density
BONE ANOMALIES non–tooth-related lesions	☐ no ☐ n/a*	☐ yes *list on reverse side*	**OTHER** ☐ n/a*	☐ document on reverse	***n/a** *cannot be determined from images reviewed; additional images needed*

ADDITIONAL NOTES

TEETH

IMPACTED TEETH			**PULP CAVITY FEATURES**	
NUMBER ANOMALIES supernumerary teeth / congenitally missing teeth				
CROWN ANOMALIES size / shape defects			**ROOT FEATURES**	
DEFECTIVE RESTORATIONS overhang / open contacts				

CARIES suspicious areas to be evaluated clinically	1		17		MISCELLANEOUS FEATURES
	2		18		
	3		19		
	4		20		
	5		21		
tooth numbers listed	6		22		
	7		23		
	8		24		
	9		25		
indicate surface	10		26		
(mesial) M	11		27		
(distal) D	12		28		
(occlusal) O	13		29		
	14		30		
	15		31		
	16		32		

BONE

PERIAPICAL AREA radiolucency			**LAMINA DURA** crestal	
PERIAPICAL AREA radiopacity			**LAMINA DURA** radicular	
BONE LOSS percent & pattern			**PDL SPACE**	
			FURCATION INVOLVEMENT	
			INTERDENTAL TRABECULATIONS	
BONE ANOMALIES non–tooth-related lesions			**OTHER**	

IMAGES NEEDED

list additional images needed	

APPLICATION

Module 7   Interpretation Basics

SELF-ASSESSMENT

Chapters 32 - 35

Based on the worksheets that you have just completed, how prepared are you for the upcoming Module 7 assessments?

_____ very prepared, confident

_____ somewhat prepared, somewhat confident

_____ somewhat unprepared, lack confidence

_____ unprepared, no confidence

Based on your answer above, what is your plan for improvement? List the topics and concepts that you need to further review and study for assessments.

_____

_____

_____

_____

_____

_____

CRITICAL THINKING QUESTIONS

What does interpretation mean to you in the dental setting? Use the questions below to help you apply the information that you have just learned. Work in pairs and practice answering these questions with your classmates. Share feedback concerning the content and delivery of information—is the information correct and understandable for the average patient? Are effective communication skills being used? The more you practice, the more comfortable you will be discussing these issues with your patients.

1. **A student at the local university has come into your office for a career day. She is interested in becoming a part of the dental team and would like to see what each job entails and what it is like to be in the dental profession for a day. As you are explaining to her the daily routine of your office, she asks who takes and who interprets dental images. How can you answer the student correctly?**

2. **After viewing a complete series of dental images, what should the dental radiographer document in the patient's record?**

TO-DO CHECKLIST

Written Exercises

_____ Complete all worksheets.

_____ Complete self-assessment.

Active Learning Experiences

_____ Complete all interpretation exercises.

_____ Review and answer the critical thinking questions.

_____ Practice answering critical thinking questions with your classmates and provide feedback.

X-radiation is harmful to living tissues. Because biologic damage results from x-ray exposure, dental images are pre-scribed for a patient only when the benefit of disease detection outweighs the risk of biologic damage. When dental images are properly prescribed and exposed, the benefit of disease detection far outweighs the risk of damage from x-radiation.

All x-radiation is harmful. To protect the patient and operator from excess radiation exposure, radiation exposure guidelines have been established. These guidelines include radiation safety legislation and exposure limits for the general public and for persons who are occupationally exposed to radiation.

In this portion of the dental radiography course, students, staff, and faculty members will be using x-radiation. Before beginning, a review of basic information on the use of ionizing radiation is necessary.

1 Use of Ionizing Radiation

RADIATION SAFETY PROCEDURES AND POLICIES

As dental radiographers, our goal is to minimize patient exposure to radiation while producing images of good diagnostic quality. All operators of dental x-ray equipment are responsible for following radiation safety procedures. The program director of the dental hygiene or dental assisting program is the radiation safety officer (RSO) unless the role is otherwise delegated to the radiology course director.

This person has the responsibility to oversee matters related to radiation protection. The RSO confirms that all training has been completed and also serves as the contact person with the state. Employees and students should submit all radiation concerns to the RSO. If suspicion of a radiation incident or accidental exposure occurs, immediately notify the RSO or department head.

Please record the name of the RSO of your institution: _____

Operation of X-Ray Equipment

Before beginning any assignments in the radiology laboratory, the following information is necessary to review:

- In the laboratory, *Never* expose anyone to ionizing radiation during laboratory procedures.
- *Never* press the exposure button unless being certain that no person is inside the radiology cubicle during laboratory procedures.
- *Do not* stand in the doorway or in the direct line of the primary beam when radiation is being produced.
- *Do not* operate the x-ray equipment unless authorized by a faculty member or dentist.
- *Only* the teaching manikin (DXTTR) is allowed in the cubicle during a radiographic examination.
  - Do not hold or stabilize the patient or teaching manikin during exposure.
  - Do not hold the image receptor (film or digital sensor) in place for a patient during exposure.
  - Do not hold or stabilize the x-ray tubehead during radiographic procedures.
- If you are working in pairs or in small groups with the teaching manikin, make certain that *all* persons have left the room before x-ray exposure.
- Utilize correct exposure settings for mA, kV, and time for each anatomic area as dictated by the settings on the exposure control panel (Fig. 1-1).
- *Do not* alter or tamper with the machines' radiation protection devices, including lead-lined position indicating devices, aluminum filters, and lead collimators.

Position and Distance Recommendations for Operators of X-Ray Equipment

Locate the safety areas discussed below in the radiology clinic of your institution.

- The dental radiographer should always stand completely behind a protective barrier; use a wall mirror or window to view the teaching manikin and patient during radiographic procedures.
- Do not stand in the path of the central beam of radiation (such as the doorway) during exposures. Always stand behind a lead barrier or proper thickness of drywall during exposures.
- Never stand closer than 6 feet to the x-ray machine during an exposure, unless standing behind a barrier or wall.
- If a wall or protective barrier is unavailable, the area outlined in gray in Fig. 1-2 is a safe place to stand.

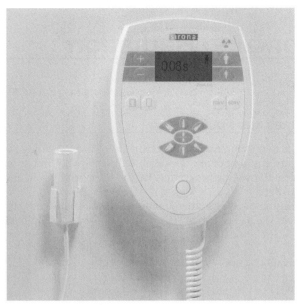

Fig. 1-1. Heliodent control panel. Courtesy of Sirona Dental Inc. USA, Charlotte, NC.

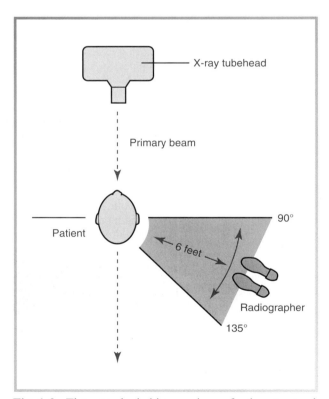

Fig. 1-2. The area shaded in gray is a safe place to stand.

Radiology Cubicles

- In areas where x-rays are being generated and imaging equipment is in use, a sign with the radiation symbol must be displayed stating, "CAUTION: X-RAYS" or "RADIATION AREA" (Fig. 1-3). Make certain this sign is visible in the radiology cubicles.

- Safety instructions should be posted or made available in the radiography area, including information on the safe operation of the equipment and emergency procedures.

- Each radiology cubicle should have its own lead apron and thyroid collar (Fig. 1-4).

  - Locate the lead aprons and thyroid collars in the radiology cubicles of your institution; notice the condition and weight of the aprons.

  - Lead aprons contain 0.25 mm or more lead equivalence. Periodically check the apron and thyroid collar for cracks, holes, or tears.

  - Use the protective lead apron *and thyroid collar* on the teaching manikin and all patients during *intraoral* radiographic procedures.

  - Use the protective lead apron (*without the thyroid collar*) on all patients during *extraoral* radiographic procedures.

  - Do not handle the lead apron with gloves; always place and remove the lead apron with clean hands only.

  - Use the hanger provided to store the lead apron properly (Fig. 1-5).

- Guidelines will be provided in the panoramic cubicle for receptor and patient positioning before exposure.

- Stand behind a protective barrier and watch the patient during panoramic exposure.

Radiation Monitoring

- Observation of all personnel who are involved with radiographic procedures (faculty, staff, and students) should be monitored with a radiation badge (dosimetry) service (Fig. 1-6), however, the dosimetry service is not required by all states.

- Each operator should wear his or her own badge and not share badges between people.

- The badge should be worn at waist level whenever working in the radiology clinic.

- Radiation badges are *not* to be worn when the operator is undergoing any radiation exposures as a patient.

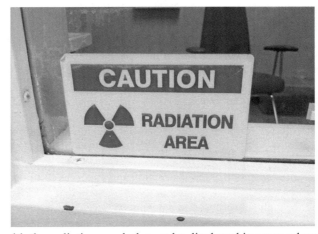

Fig. 1-3. A sign with the radiation symbol must be displayed in areas where x-rays are in use.

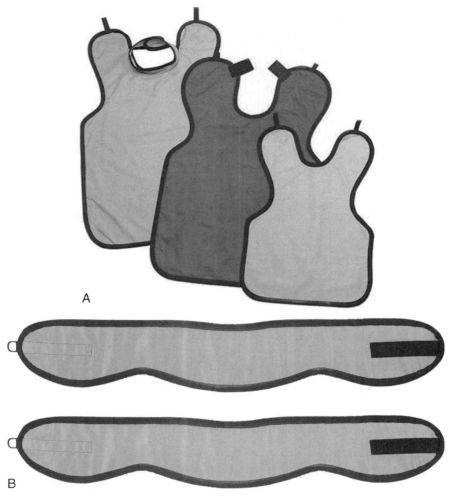

Fig. 1-4. A, Lead aprons with thyroid collars. **B,** Thyroid collars. Courtesy of DUX Dental, Oxnard, CA.

- Tampering with or use of radiation badges for any purposes other than those intended will not be tolerated.

- Records of radiation exposures should be kept on file in the administrative office.

Responsibilities

It is the responsibility of the *teaching institution* to do the following:
- Maintain the dental radiation equipment and comply with state regulations for protection against radiation.

- Request annual inspection of radiation equipment.

- Designate a qualified Radiation Safety Officer to coordinate maintenance of equipment and instruction in utilizing dental radiation.

- Provide faculty who have current credentials in the instruction and supervision of dental radiology procedures.

- Provide personnel monitoring through subscription to a dosimetry service.

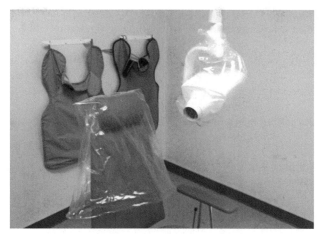

Fig. 1-5. Lead aprons are stored properly on hangers.

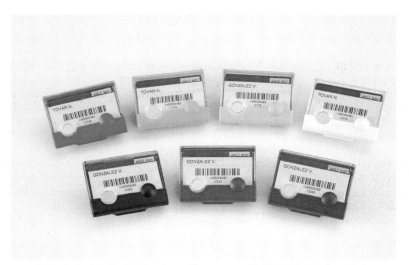

Fig. 1-6. Radiation badges. Courtesy of ICCARE, Irvine, CA.

It is the responsibility of the *faculty* to do the following:

- Ensure that dentists prescribe images that are diagnostically necessary for complete patient care.

- Provide instruction and evaluation through a didactic radiology course, including laboratory competencies, with the use of a teaching manikin.

- Ensure that images prescribed are exposed with the permission of the patient.

- Monitor any retakes that may be needed.

- Oversee that images are exposed in an efficient, timely, and compassionate manner.

- Confirm that all quality assurance protocol is implemented, maintained, and documented including all darkroom and processing procedures, digital imaging equipment, and dosimetry badge readings.

- Review and grade all images and competency examinations, providing remediation when necessary.

It is the responsibility of the *student* to do the following:

- Follow all protocol for radiation safety in laboratory and clinical assignments.

- Expose images of patients for diagnostic purposes only; the images must be prescribed by a licensed dentist.

  o Additional exposures are never exposed to improve a grade or achieve a competency level.

- Ensure the exercises with the teaching manikin are handled in the same manner as the procedures used with a clinical patient.

- When treating patients in the clinical setting, document patient permission for imaging procedures along with medical and dental histories and other necessary demographic information.

- Complete the proper exposure of the images (teaching manikin or patient) using proper infection control procedures and radiographic technique in a timely manner.

- Seek remediation by faculty when necessary.

Time in the Radiology Laboratory

Policies and procedures in the laboratory can vary by institution and instructor, but the following are best practices:
Most of the time in the radiology laboratory will be spent learning and practicing the various intraoral and extraoral techniques that will be used in clinical situations. Some laboratory exercises are easily accomplished and may go quickly, whereas others may present more challenging scenarios and warrant extra time. Either way, it is strongly recommended to leave the radiology clinic area clean and stocked full of supplies before departing at the end of the laboratory session.

Regardless of the way the room was left before your laboratory experience, take the extra effort to clean and disinfect the radiology cubicles and surrounding work areas. Wipe down sink and countertop areas; leave the dental chair in a comfortable working position, and place the x-ray tubehead firmly against the wall. No signs of debris or glove dust should be visible on the lead apron. If the trash can is full, discard it appropriately and replace with a clean trash bag liner. Stock all supplies, including personal protective equipment and radiology work items. Turn off the x-ray machine and overhead lights if appropriate.

These efforts do not go unnoticed and will go a long way, especially when an operator is in a difficult position while working with a patient. If everyone pitches in and does more than their "fair share," the environment in the radiology clinic will be positive and welcoming.

Make good use of all of your time in the radiology laboratory!

Name _____

Date _____

ASSESSMENT 1-1

Radiation Safety Procedures and Policies

1. Describe and identify the parts of the radiation badges used in your institution.

_____

_____

_____

2. What type of questions may the patient ask when seeing the radiology caution sign?

_____

_____

_____

3. During x-ray exposures, is it safe to stand outside of the radiology cubicle in the doorway? Why or why not?

_____

_____

_____

4. What construction materials are included inside the walls of the radiology cubicle at your institution?

_____

_____

_____

2 | Equipment Used in the Radiology Clinic

INSIDE THE RADIOLOGY CUBICLE

X-Ray Machine
The x-ray machine (Fig. 2-1) features three parts:
- The exposure control panel (A) is in a radiation-safe area outside of the cubicle.
- The extension arm (B) and tubehead (C) are both found inside the radiology cubicle.

Control Panel
- The on/off switch for the x-ray machine is usually located on the underside of the control panel, fixed to the wall.
- Look for a light on the panel that indicates if the machine is on or off. The arrow points to a green light, signaling that the x-ray machine is "on" (Fig. 2-2).
- Once the machine is turned on, the exposure control panel on the outside of the radiology cubicle will also be illuminated.

Extension Arm
- The arm contains electrical wires and allows for movement and positioning of the tubehead.
- The mechanical support of the x-ray tubehead and position indicating device (PID) should maintain the exposure position without drift or vibration.
- It is recommended to store the tubehead against the wall, PID pointed downward, as shown in Fig. 2-3. Check with the faculty regarding correct storage of the x-ray machine particular to your facility.
  - Adjust the extension arm so it is also against the wall with arms folded as close together as possible.
  - Leaving an x-ray machine out or suspended near the dental chair will cause the extension arm to become loose and may produce more drifting of the x-ray tubehead.

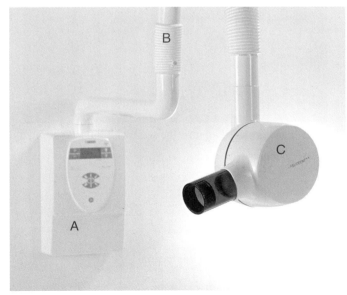

Fig. 2-1. Three component parts of dental x-ray machine. **A,** Control panel. **B,** Extension arm. **C,** Tubehead. Courtesy Sirona Dental USA Inc., Charlotte, NC.

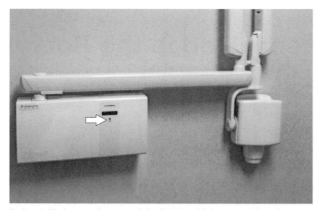

Fig. 2-2. A light on the panel indicates if the machine is on or off.

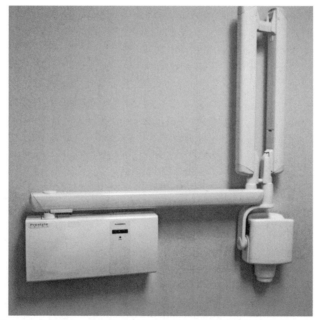

Fig. 2-3. The tubehead is stored against the wall with the PID pointed downward.

Tubehead

- The tubehead houses the dental x-ray tube (Fig. 2-4).

- The PID extends from the tubehead and directs the x-ray beam.

  o The PID is circular or rectangular in shape, with a lead lining.

  o This is the location where the central or primary beam of the x-ray beam exits the tubehead.

  o Verify which type of PID is found in the radiology cubicles; ie, whether it is round or rectangular.

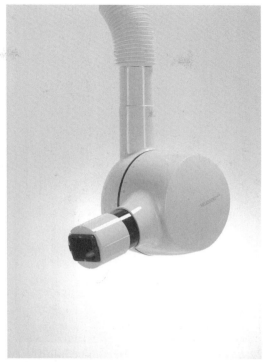

Fig. 2-4. The tubehead contains the x-ray tube. Courtesy of Sirona Dental Inc. USA, Charlotte, NC.

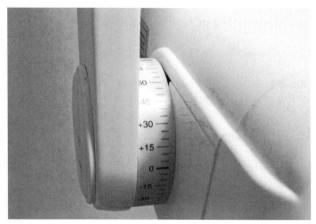

Fig. 2-5. The numbered dial shows vertical angulation in degrees.

- The tubehead is an expensive piece of equipment, therefore it should always be handled carefully.

  o Do not make sudden movements with the extension arm or force the machine into an awkward position at any time.

- On the side of the tubehead is a numbered dial that measures vertical angulation (positive and negative) in degrees (Fig. 2-5).

- Vertical angulation refers to the positioning of the PID in a vertical plane.

  o Most maxillary periapical images will be produced with the tubehead pointing downward, which is a *positive* vertical angulation.

  o Most mandibular periapical images will be produced with the tubehead angled slightly upward, which is a *negative* vertical angulation.

329

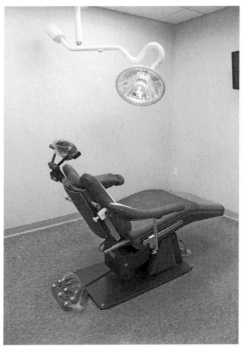

Fig. 2-6. Dental chair. Copyright lutherhill/Istock.com.

- Horizontal angulation refers to the positioning of the PID in a horizontal plane.

  ○ The horizontal angulation can also be changed by moving the tubehead (not the extension arm) from side to side.

- Choosing the correct horizontal angulation will be an important concept in the production of diagnostic images and will be better understood once the intraoral radiology techniques are learned.

Dental (Patient) Chair
- The dental chair is for the patient or teaching manikin to sit (Fig. 2-6).

- The height of the chair should be positioned so that it is comfortable for the operator to access all sides of the patient (front, back, right, and left) during radiographic procedures.

- The tubehead should be able to reach all sides of the patient without the operator having to strain or exert effort. The dental chair may also rotate or turn from side to side, if tubehead access is limited.

- Most intraoral images are exposed with the patient seated upright so that the patient occlusal plane is parallel to the floor.

- The back of the dental chair should be positioned so the patient sits straight during radiographic procedures, and the headrest should be adjusted for support.

  ○ Encourage use of the headrest for stabilization during x-ray exposures, which will diminish the chance for patient movement.

Lead Apron and Thyroid Collar
- A lead apron and thyroid collar are used for patient protection during intraoral exposures (Fig. 2-7).

- Use of the lead apron and thyroid collar is mandatory for all patients but is also recommended for the teaching manikin, aiding the student into its routine use.

330

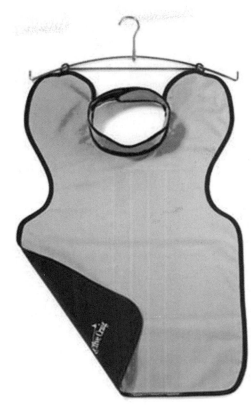

Fig. 2-7. Lead apron with collar. Courtesy of DUX Dental, Oxnard, CA.

- ○ The apron is laid over the front of the patient and usually attached behind the neck with Velcro straps.

- ○ The thyroid collar should be placed around the neck of the patient, again adhering in back.

- Although bulky and cumbersome, the lead apron should be handled with care with clean hands only. The lead apron is not able to be heat sterilized so clean hands *(no gloves!)* are recommended for handling.

- Proper storage of lead protective aprons prolongs their life and effectiveness.

  - ○ Aprons should be hung straight (instead of folded) because creases may eventually become cracks that can allow radiation to penetrate.

  - ○ Do not lay the apron over the dental chair when not in use.

Dental X-Ray Teaching and Training Manikin (DXTTR)

The dental x-ray teaching manikin (Fig. 2-8) is a realistic substitute to allow instruction of various types of intraoral radiographic techniques. According to the manufacturer (Dentsply RINN), mechanical operations and components of the teaching manikin are designed for durability, ease of use, lifelike movements, and adjustment features.

- The teaching manikin is referred to as "DXTTR," which refers to Dental x-ray Training and Teaching Replica." DXTTR is used for intraoral radiology exercises and is usually kept inside the radiology cubicle in a drawer or cabinet.

- DXTTR will serve as the "patient" for all practice exercises in this portion of the dental radiography course. All exposed images completed during the laboratory portion of the radiography course will be completed with the teaching manikin. Again, ensure that *no* student, staff, or faculty member is inside the radiology cubicle during exposures.

- Please note that the training manikin *must be handled with care!* The manikin is subject to high stress and should be properly used and safely stored. Teeth may be prone to breakage and the outer facial skin may be torn. The jaws articulate mechanically, but closing mechanisms may wear and not allow the teeth to occlude completely.

331

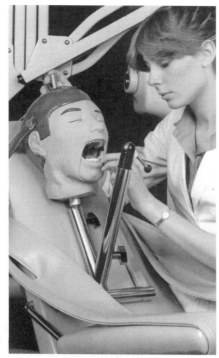

Fig. 2-8. DXTTR Teaching Manikin placed in a chair. Courtesy of Dentsply Rinn Corporation, York, PA.

- Carefully place the manikin in the dental chair and secure it with two hooks to the back of the dental chair. An adjustable nylon strap will hold the manikin head securely in place against the headrest of the chair. Clamp the lever underneath the chin to support the head securely in position.

- Because repairs and refurbishment of the teaching manikin are costly, make certain that it is handled carefully and stored correctly after each use.

- If you notice any part of DXTTR malfunctioning, notify the instructor immediately.

Computer Equipment
Depending on the type of digital imaging equipment used, a computer, keyboard, mouse, and monitor may also be located inside the radiology cubicle.
- Manufacturer's instructions should be followed for correct handling and infection control for this equipment.

- A protective barrier fits snugly over the keyboard inside the radiology cubicle (Fig. 2-9). The mouse also requires a plastic cover.

Miscellaneous Supplies
Other supplies usually found inside the x-ray cubicle include a sink with antiseptic soap for hand washing as well as a supply of gloves and masks. A sanitizing hand gel may also be in a dispensing unit.
    An area with hooks for patient coats or handbags is optional but convenient.
Additional supplies that may be helpful for the operator include:
- cotton rolls, gauze squares, and tongue depressors (Fig. 2-10)

- soft foam cushions for the corners of receptors provide a more comfortable edge and may be needed for those patients who have difficulty biting down completely (Fig. 2-11)

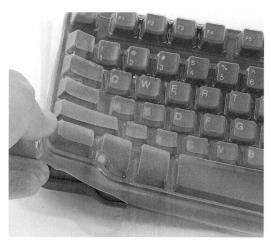

Fig. 2-9. Keyboard cover. Courtesy of Medicus Health, Kentworth, MI.

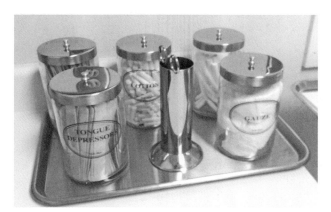

Fig. 2-10. Miscellaneous supplies on a tray.

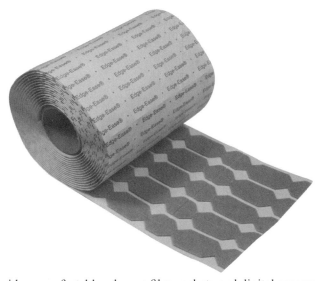

Fig. 2-11. Foam cushions provide a comfortable edge on film packets and digital sensors. (Photo courtesy Patterson Dental, St. Paul, MN)

333

Name _____

Date _____

ASSESSMENT 2-1

Inside the Radiology Cubicle

1. Are any items visible inside the radiology cubicle that may make a patient nervous? If so, what steps would be necessary to manage an anxious patient before radiographic procedures?

_____

_____

_____

2. A patient complains that the lead apron and thyroid collar are too heavy and uncomfortable. What would be an appropriate response?

_____

_____

_____

3. The teaching manikin is older and will not stay closed when locking its jaws. What would be an appropriate solution?

_____

_____

_____

4. An intraoral receptor is placed and the PID is aligned correctly. Upon exiting the cubicle to depress the exposure button, the operator notices that the machine is not turned on. What is the appropriate next step?

_____

_____

_____

5. What is the problem with a tubehead that drifts? What errors may result on the dental images?

_____

_____

_____

X-Ray Machine Exposure Control Panel

The exposure control panel (Fig. 2-12) is in a radiation-safe area outside of the cubicle.

* The on/off switch for the x-ray machine is usually located on the underside of the panel fixed to the wall *inside* the radiology cubicle. Look for a light on the panel that indicates if the machine is on or off. Once the machine is turned on, the exposure control panel on the outside of the radiology cubicle will also be illuminated.

* The x-ray exposure control panel will illuminate once the x-ray machine is turned on.

* Various settings are available that control the intensity of the x-ray beam and the amount of x-radiation produced.

* Some dental units have predetermined programmable settings for the various anatomic areas of the oral cavity. Other units must be set each time a different area of the mouth is exposed to radiation.

    o Most newer dental x-ray machines are equipped with preset programmable settings for the anatomic areas of the maxilla and mandible.

    o The manufacturer of the dental x-ray machine has determined an "average" setting for the anterior teeth, premolar and molar areas, and different settings for the maxilla and mandible.

    o The timer is electronically controlled to provide exact exposure time in fractions of a second, or impulses.

    o Older units may require that the operator choose the correct kilovoltage, milliamperage and time controls setting for each exposure.

Remember:

* The kilovoltage controls the penetrating power of the x-ray beam (usually set between 65 and 100 kV)

* The milliamperage (mA) controls the amount of electrons passing through the cathode. Increased mA results in the production of an increased number of x-rays.

* Exposure time, as with milliamperage, controls the number of x-rays produced. A longer exposure time produces more x-rays.

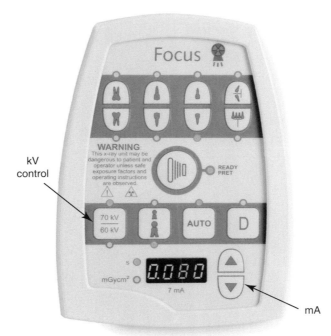

Fig. 2-12. Exposure control panel. Courtesy Instrumentarium Dental, Inc., Milwaukee, WI.

Depending on the clinic area, a single, centrally located control panel may be used to operate several x-ray machines located in separate treatment rooms. Although not recommended, the radiology treatment rooms may have been constructed this way to save space.

Exposure Button/Switch

The exposure button (or switch) activates the x-ray machine to produce x-radiation (Fig. 2-13).

- It is extremely important to concentrate on the exposure button each time the operator leaves the radiology cubicle to make an exposure. Do not get distracted or sidetracked when operating the exposure button.

- You should always hear a "beep" and see an illuminated light indicating that an exposure has occurred. If the hallway outside the radiology cubicle is noisy or congested, the operator must listen carefully to ensure that the exposure has been made. It is unacceptable to return to the patient and ask if the machine made a beeping noise.

- The x-ray machine must have a device to terminate the exposure after a preset time; this is usually in the form of a "dead man"–type exposure switch. This type of switch requires constant pressure from the operator in order for the machine to function but will not "overexpose" a receptor.

  - **Remember**: The operator can potentially underexpose a receptor, but due to the function of the dead man switch, *the receptor should never be overexposed to radiation.*

- It is also recommended to depress the exposure button with a firm finger or thumb each time.

- If the exposure button becomes wet from patient saliva or blood, it could become slippery and cause the finger of the operator to slide off the exposure button. This could result in unnecessary radiation exposure of the patient and should be avoided.

Portable Tray/Work Area

Outside of the radiology cubicle and away from any radiation exposure is the location of a work area to keep the unexposed receptors, beam alignment devices, plastic cup with exposed receptors, cotton rolls, and any other equipment that may be needed during the radiographic examination.

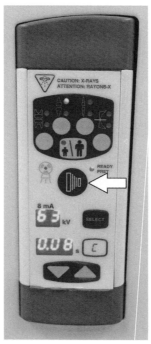

Fig. 2-13. The exposure button (*arrow*) activates the x-ray machine to produce x-radiation.

338

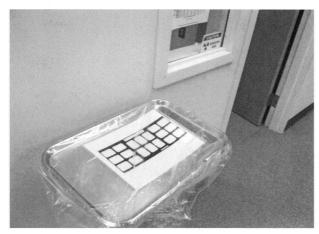

Fig. 2-14. A portable tray covered with a plastic bag; a laminated image mount is inserted beneath the plastic barrier to organize the receptors for each patient's radiographic prescription.

- Many institutions use a portable type of tray that can be covered with a plastic bag and rolled back and forth easily (Fig. 2-14). The location of the tray is just outside the radiology cubicle, enabling the operator to see the patient through the window while pressing the exposure button.

- Other facilities may have a permanent shelf designated as a radiation-safe area to work and arrange supplies.

- Organizing the prescribed receptors on top of the laminated mount is a simple way to make the radiology procedures flow easier. It also helps reduce the risk of contamination by containing all supplies in one spot, therefore eliminating the need to run back and forth between clinic areas.

Infection Control Supplies and Miscellaneous Supplies

In most institutions, a central supply area is located near the radiology treatment rooms to stock supplies needed for procedures. This may include personal protective equipment (PPE) such as gloves, masks, gowns, protective eyewear, or disinfecting solutions. Sinks for handwashing may be located inside or outside of the radiology cubicle. Other supplies required for radiographic examinations may also be located in one area, including cotton rolls, bite blocks, bite tabs, cups, foam edges or corners, gauze, topical anesthetic spray, tongue blades, and facial tissue. Be certain to follow infection control guidelines when retrieving supplies for patient care. Module 3 of this section discusses infection control in more detail.

ASSESSMENT 2-2

Outside the Radiology Cubicle

1. Demonstrate the differences between the exposure settings for anterior and posterior periapical images, as well as bite-wing images.

   _____

   _____

   _____

2. In exposing a complete mouth series, you are interrupted in the middle of the procedure. You are uncertain whether or not an exposure was made on a posterior periapical receptor because you did not hear a "beep." What is the correct course of action?

   _____

   _____

   _____

3. In exposing a complete mouth series, you accidentally drop an exposed receptor off the portable work tray. What is the correct course of action?

   _____

   _____

   _____

4. Your patient is scheduled for exposure of four bite-wing images. He is a member of the college football team and is quite tall and muscular. Should you use the preset exposure settings on the x-ray control panel? Why or why not?

   _____

   _____

   _____

IMAGE RETRIEVAL AREAS

Because not all teaching institutions are the same, some schools may primarily use traditional film, digital imaging, or a combination of both techniques. Therefore basic concepts for all image retrieval techniques will be presented.

Darkroom

X-ray film is very sensitive to light; therefore it should only be unwrapped in a darkened environment. Otherwise the image will be ruined. The darkroom is the safe location where traditional x-ray film can be opened, handled, and processed to produce diagnostic radiographs. The darkroom has been constructed to be completely light-tight, excluding all visible white light. Inside the darkroom, close the door with all the lights turned off. You should not see any extraneous light entering from the door, vent, or keyhole.

The darkroom should have two types of lighting within:
- overhead light

- safelight (Fig. 2-15)

Find the location of the switches for both the overhead light and the safelight. It is recommended not to have these light switches too close in proximity if possible. Make certain that in a darkened room, you can tell the difference between the overhead light switch and the switch for the safelight.

Darkroom doors may or may not include a lock. If your darkroom door cannot be locked from the inside, some indication that a person is working inside the darkroom must be visible from outside. In some darkrooms, turning on the safelight may also turn on an indicator light on the *outside* of the darkroom (Fig. 2-16). When illuminated, this light informs other personnel that someone is working inside the darkroom and the door is *not* to be opened! Again, remember that dental x-ray film is extremely sensitive to light.

Because x-ray film is sensitive to light, the processing solutions must be located inside the darkroom. Either manual tanks or an automatic processor (or both) will be located inside the darkroom. Busier schools with larger patient populations may require several processing machines located inside the darkroom.

Automatic processing machines can be found inside the darkroom. In addition, a daylight loader device (Fig. 2-17) may be attached to an automatic processing machine that eliminates the need for a darkroom; the film is unwrapped within the daylight loader that is constructed to be light-tight.

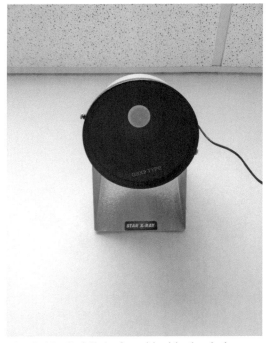

Fig. 2-15. Safelight found inside the darkroom.

A few reminders about loading x-ray film into the automatic processor:

- Make certain that only the film is inserted into the processor. The black paper, lead foil, and outer package wrapper should *not* be placed into the processor.

- Do not place films into the processor *too close together*. On average, three to four films may be placed into the processor at the film feed slot at a time.

- Many automatic processors produce a "click" noise when it is safe to place additional films into the processor.

- Make certain that the rollers take and pull the film into the processor. Do not simply lay the film at the film feed slot alone.

It may help to practice loading unexposed films into the automatic processor in a lighted room first, followed by developing DXTTR films under the safelight conditions. These same guidelines pertain to the daylight loader device, as it is also attached to the top of an automatic processor.

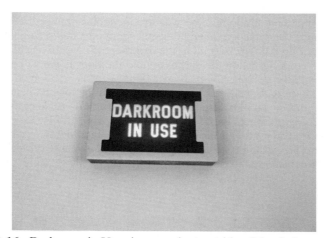

Fig. 2-16. Darkroom in Use sign seen just outside of the darkroom door.

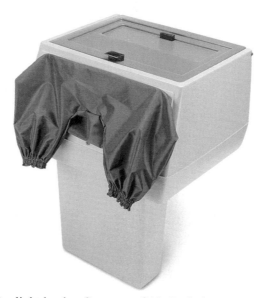

Fig. 2-17. Daylight loader. Courtesy of Air Techniques Inc., Melville, NY.

Digital Imaging

Many institutions offer some form of digital imaging for patient care. Digital imaging is preferred over traditional x-ray film because less radiation is needed to produce an image. Less radiation for the patient follows the ALARA Principle, in keeping all radiation doses "as low as reasonably achievable."

Two types of digital imaging are commonly used in dentistry:

- *Direct digital imaging* refers to a system that places a wired sensor inside the patient's mouth, exposes it to radiation, and transmits the image to a computer monitor within moments.

- *Indirect digital imaging* refers to a system that places a sensor inside the patient's mouth, exposes it to radiation, and uses a high-speed scanning device to convert the digital data into an image on the computer monitor.

Images produced with direct and indirect digital imaging procedures are viewed on the computer monitor. Some computer monitors are located within the radiology cubicle, whereas others may be found at each operatory for patient care.

Direct Digital Imaging

The pieces of equipment needed for direct digital imaging systems include an x-ray machine, a wired intraoral sensor, and a computer monitor. Only one sensor, which is placed into the patient's mouth for each exposure, is used in this type of digital imaging (Fig. 2-18). Once exposed to radiation, the image appears on the computer monitor. The image on the sensor is automatically cleared, and the same sensor is then ready for additional exposures.

Infection control is very important in direct digital imaging because the sensor cannot withstand heat sterilization. Because the same sensor is used for all patients, the possibility increases for cross-contamination to occur. The sensor and portions of the wire attachment must be wrapped with a disposable plastic sleeve (Fig. 2-19). A disinfecting solution wipe may also be required for the direct digital sensor.

Indirect Digital Imaging

The equipment needed for indirect digital imaging systems include an x-ray machine, intraoral sensors (phosphor plates), a laser scanning device, and a computer monitor. Intraoral sensors are individually wrapped in plastic barrier envelopes, similar to traditional film. Just like film, each sensor is exposed in various anatomic regions of the mouth. When all phosphor plates have been exposed, the plates are unwrapped and placed into a laser scanning device (Fig. 2-20). The scanning device records the diagnostic data from the plates and converts it into electronic files to be seen on the computer monitor. Before the plates can be reused, the data must be erased.

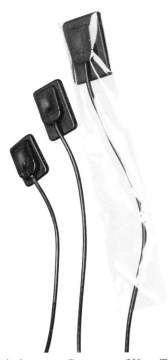

Fig. 2-18. Wired digital sensor. Courtesy of Kerr TotalCare, Orange, CA.

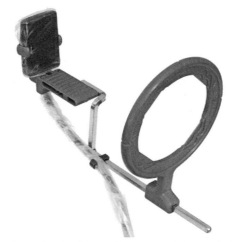

Fig. 2-19. The sensor in a plastic sleeve. Courtesy of Dentsply Rinn Corp., York, PA.

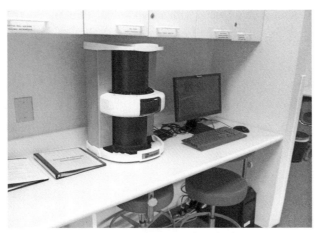

Fig. 2-20. Laser scanning device.

ASSESSMENT 2-3

Image Retrieval Areas

1. List the four items that make-up an x-ray film packet. Now, closing your eyes, can you unwrap a film packet and identify which component is the actual film?

   _____

   _____

   _____

2. In the darkroom, how far away from the work surface is the location of the safelight? Why?

   _____

   _____

   _____

3. If your institution uses intraoral digital imaging, identify the type(s): direct or indirect?

   _____

   _____

   _____

4. If your institution uses extraoral digital imaging, identify the type(s): direct or indirect?

   _____

   _____

   _____

5. What may be the result of films placed too close together into the automatic processor?

   _____

   _____

   _____

6. How close in proximity are the switches for the darkroom overhead light and the safelight? Are these switches easy to identify in a darkened room?

   _____

   _____

   _____

CLINICAL LABORATORY ACTIVITY 2-1

Inside the Radiation Cubicle

Objectives

- Identify the component parts of the dental x-ray machine.

- Demonstrate how to turn the machine on and off; verify when the machine is on.

- Demonstrate a PID with both positive and negative vertical angulations.

- Demonstrate a PID with various horizontal angulations.

- Discuss the correct position of the dental chair during radiographic procedures.

- Locate and identify any computer equipment and miscellaneous supplies found inside the radiology cubicle.

Introduction

The goal of this laboratory exercise is to familiarize the student with the location and operation of the dental x-ray equipment found inside the radiology cubicle.

Procedure

1. Wash hands and prepare with proper PPE.

2. Review all pieces of equipment found inside the radiology cubicle and discuss their functions.

Name _____

Date _____

CLINICAL LABORATORY ACTIVITY 2-1 WORKSHEET

Perform each task in the Equipment List, recording your comments in the space provided.

Equipment List and Function	Completed (✓)	Student Comments
X-ray machine on/off switch • Demonstrate proper use • Verify with lighted exposure control panel outside of cubicle		
Extension arm • Discuss its importance and proper storage between use		
Tubehead • Demonstrate the aiming of the central ray and importance of the PID • Identify round or rectangular collimation		
Vertical angulation PID • Demonstrate positive and negative vertical angulation		
Horizontal angulation PID • Demonstrate changing horizontal angulation		
Dental chair position • Discuss proper chair position for operator and patient • Demonstrate various chair positions • Ensure that the tubehead can access all sides of the dental chair		
Lead apron and thyroid collar • Demonstrate proper way to place on a patient • Demonstrate proper way to store lead apron and thyroid collar		
Teaching manikin • Discuss proper way to handle the manikin, set it up, and store it correctly		
Computer equipment • If applicable, demonstrate correct ways to turn on computer and begin software programs for radiography		
Infection control supplies • Demonstrate location of gloves, masks, sanitary wipes, cotton rolls, handwashing supplies, and all infection control supplies		
Miscellaneous supplies • Demonstrate location of any other supplies in the radiology cubicle that may be necessary during radiographic procedures		

Faculty Signature: _____ **Date:** _____

CLINICAL LABORATORY ACTIVITY 2-2

Outside the Radiation Cubicle

Objectives

- Identify the component parts of the x-ray exposure control panel.

- Demonstrate how to adjust settings for kilovoltage, milliamperage, and time.

- Demonstrate correct settings for various sizes and anatomic areas of patients.

- Demonstrate the correct way to make an exposure.

- List the common items found on the portable tray.

Introduction

The goal of this laboratory exercise is to familiarize the student with the location and operation of the dental x-ray equipment found outside of the radiology cubicle.

Procedure

1. Wash hands and prepare with proper PPE.

2. Review all equipment found outside the radiology cubicle.

Name _____

Date _____

CLINICAL LABORATORY ACTIVITY 2-2 WORKSHEET

Perform each task in the Equipment List, recording your comments in the space provided.

Equipment List and Function	Completed (✓)	Student Comments
X-ray machine on/off switch • Demonstrate proper use • Verify with lighted exposure control panel outside of cubicle		
X-ray exposure control panel • Demonstrate various settings for different anatomic regions • Demonstrate changing kV, mA, or time settings		
Exposure button • Demonstrate correct way to make an exposure • Demonstrate an "underexposure"		
Portable tray or work area • List equipment which should be located in this radiation-safe area		
Infection control supplies • Demonstrate location of gloves, masks, sanitary wipes, cotton rolls, handwashing supplies, and all infection control supplies		
Miscellaneous supplies • Demonstrate location of any other supplies outside the radiology cubicle that may be necessary during radiographic procedures		

Faculty Signature: _____   **Date:** _____

CLINICAL LABORATORY ACTIVITY 2-3

Image Retrieval Areas

Objectives

- Identify the equipment and location of the darkroom; discuss the size, lighting, processing, and equipment requirements.

- Examine and observe the function of the daylight loader machine.

- Describe the type of equipment needed for direct digital imaging procedures.

- Describe the type of equipment needed for indirect digital imaging procedures.

Introduction

The goal of this laboratory exercise is to familiarize the student with the location and operation of the dental x-ray equipment found in the image retrieval areas. This may include the darkroom, daylight loader, scanning area, or other areas where computer access is available.

Step-by-Step Procedure

1. Wash hands and prepare with proper PPE.

2. Prepare radiology cubicle with appropriate infection control protocol.

3. Set up the training manikin and utilize lead apron and thyroid collar.

4. Turn on the x-ray machine and set to the exposure setting of the maxillary canine.

5. Retrieve receptors in a plastic cup and place on the work area just outside the radiology cubicle.

6. Expose receptors in the anterior maxilla using film, direct digital imaging, or indirect digital imaging. (If using direct digital imaging, images will be viewed immediately after exposure on the computer monitor in the radiology cubicle.)

7. Once all exposures are complete, remove gloves, wash hands, and proceed to the image retrieval areas.

Name _____

Date _____

Upon reviewing equipment in image retrieval areas, inform faculty to check that all items have been identified correctly.

Item	Equipment Identified (✓)	Student Comments
Darkroom lighting		
Darkroom processor		
Daylight loader		
Computer equipment		
Direct digital imaging sensor		
Indirect digital imaging sensor		
Laser scanning device		
Miscellaneous equipment		

Faculty Signature: _____   **Date:** _____

3 Infection Control Procedures in the Radiology Clinic

PREVENTING THE TRANSMISSION OF INFECTION

To protect both themselves and patients, dental professionals must understand and use infection control protocols. The primary purpose of infection control procedures is to prevent the transmission of pathogens and infectious diseases. In dentistry, disease transmission may occur as a result of one of the following:
1. direct contact with pathogens in saliva, blood, respiratory secretions, or lesions
2. indirect contact with contaminated objects or instruments
3. direct contact with airborne contaminants present in spatter or aerosols, or oral and respiratory fluids

Any of the three conditions above may occur in the radiology clinic!

For infection to occur, the conditions that must be present include the following:
- a susceptible host
- a pathogen with sufficient infectivity and numbers to cause infections, and
- a portal of entry for the pathogen to infect the host

NOTE: The Centers for Disease Control and Prevention (CDC) Universal Precautions state that all blood, bodily fluids, or other potentially infectious materials should be treated as infectious. Although many dental radiographic procedures do not directly involve exposure to blood, *the presence of saliva may be enough to require adherence to the standard.*

Sterilization of Instruments

The CDC classifies dental instruments and equipment into three categories. Disinfection guidelines vary based on the risk of transmitting infectious agents.
- **Critical instruments:** Instruments that are used to penetrate soft tissue or bone must be sterilized after each use.
  - Examples include forceps, scalpels, bone chisels, scalers, and surgical burs.
  - In dental imaging, no critical instruments are used.
- **Semicritical instruments:** Instruments that contact but do not penetrate soft tissue or bone must also be sterilized after each use.
  - If the instrument can be damaged by heat and sterilization is not feasible, high-level disinfection is required.
  - Beam alignment devices, bite guides, and intraoral receptors are examples of semicritical instruments used in dental imaging (Fig. 3-1).
  - Check with manufacturers recommendations for disinfection of digital imaging equipment.
- **Noncritical instruments:** This includes instruments or devices that do not come in contact with mucous membranes. Because little risk of transmitting infection from noncritical devices exists, intermediate-level or low-level infection techniques are required for their care between patients.
  - In dental imaging, include the position indicating device (PID), the dental x-ray tubehead, x-ray arm the exposure button, the x-ray control panel (Fig. 3-2), and the lead apron; with digital imaging, include the computer keyboard and mouse.

Because radiographic procedures do not require the use of critical instruments, it may not seem to be an infectious event; however, the activities involved in dental radiographic procedures provide opportunities for cross-contamination. Infection control procedures must be adhered to carefully.

The Centers for Disease Control Guidelines for Infection Control in Dental Health Care Settings (2003) outlines specific infection control measures that pertain to dentistry, including personal protective equipment (PPE), hand hygiene, and sterilization or disinfection of instruments. The recommended infection control practices are applicable to all settings in which dental treatment is provided. The same infection control procedures must be used for each patient, with no exceptions and no extra precautions for select patients.

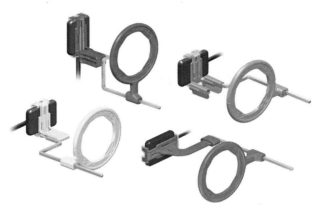

Fig. 3-1. Beam alignment devices are a type of semicritical instrument. Courtesy Dentsply Rinn Corp., York, PA.

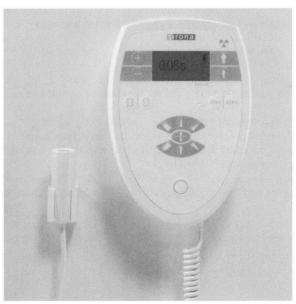

Fig. 3-2. The exposure switch and control panel are noncritical instruments.

ASSESSMENT 3-1

Preventing the Transmission of Infection

1. What are some common infections that one may encounter when working closely with other students?

   _____

   _____

   _____

2. With regard to infection control procedures, how does the radiology cubicle compare to other patient treatment rooms?

   _____

   _____

   _____

3. What clinic scenario may require a critical instrument being brought into the radiology cubicle area?

   _____

   _____

   _____

4. The intraoral placement of a mandibular anterior receptor has irritated the floor of the mouth of the patient, causing it to bleed. What procedures should be altered to protect against the spatter of blood?

   _____

   _____

   _____

5. Compared to intraoral radiography, are infection control procedures as strict during extraoral imaging?

   _____

   _____

   _____

6. Compared to intraoral radiography, are infection control procedures as strict during extraoral imaging? What infection control steps are important for panoramic exposures?

   _____

   _____

   _____

CLINICAL LABORATORY ACTIVITY 3-1

Prepare the Unit for Patient Care

Objectives

- Describe the rationale for infection control.

- Define the terms critical, semicritical, and noncritical; identify instruments used in the radiology treatment area into one of these categories.

- Use PPE in the radiology treatment area.

- Practice infection control procedures in the radiology treatment area.

Introduction

The goal of this laboratory activity is to become familiar with radiology infection control procedures. This includes infection control procedures used before, during, and after radiation exposures. The student must understand infection control procedures and their importance before beginning assignments in the radiology laboratory.

Equipment Needed

- PPE, including protective attire, gloves, mask, and eye protection

- individual radiation badge

- disposable materials including plastic wrap, plastic bags, or aluminum foil for wrapping

- disposable waste area

- disinfecting solutions

- autoclave and sterilization bags, sterilization supplies

- teaching manikin

Procedure

1. Wash hands and prepare with proper PPE. Make certain radiation badge is worn and visible.

2. In each radiology cubicle, disinfect wipe, and cover all areas that may be contacted during radiographic procedures. This includes the x-ray machine, control panel, and exposure button; the dental chair and adjustment controls; the work area where receptors are placed; any portable trays or countertops; and the keyboard, mouse, and other devices used with digital imaging. *Take caution when spraying near electrical outlets.*

3. The lead apron should also be disinfected by wiping it thoroughly.

4. Once all areas are properly prepared, seat the patient (teaching manikin).

5. Wash hands and place the lead apron on the manikin.

6. After completion, obtain a faculty signature for correct completion of infection control procedures.

Name _____

Date _____

CLINICAL LABORATORY ACTIVITY 3-1 WORKSHEET

Upon completion of Clinical Activity 3-1, place a check mark (✓) next to each item listed, identifying the radiology equipment as either a critical, semicritical or noncritical instrument. Ask your instructor to check that all infection control procedures have been prepared correctly on the equipment.

ITEM	CRITICAL	SEMICRITICAL	NONCRITICAL	INFECTION CONTROL CORRECT AND COMPLETE (✓)
X-ray machine and PID (Courtesy Sirona USA, Charlotte, NC.)				
Control panel, exposure button (Courtesy Sirona USA, Charlotte, NC.)				
Patient chair (Copyright lutherhill/iStock.com.)				

ITEM	CRITICAL	SEMICRITICAL	NONCRITICAL	INFECTION CONTROL CORRECT AND COMPLETE (✓)
Portable tray for receptors				
Lead apron (Courtesy DUX Dental, Oxnard, CA.)				
Image receptor (Courtesy Gail F. Williamson, Indianapolis, IN.)				
Beam alignment devices (Courtesy Dentsply Rinn, York, PA.)				

Module **3** **Infection Control Procedures in the Radiology Clinic**

ITEM	CRITICAL	SEMICRITICAL	NONCRITICAL	INFECTION CONTROL CORRECT AND COMPLETE (✓)
Bite blocks (Courtesy Dentsply Rinn, York, PA.)				
Receptor transfer cup (Copyright Devonyu/iStock.com)				
Computer equipment				

Faculty Signature: _____   **Date:** _____

CLINICAL LABORATORY ACTIVITY 3-2

During and After Exposures

Objectives

- Discuss the appropriate infection control procedures used during and after x-ray exposures.

- Discuss ways to minimize contamination during exposures.

- Demonstrate the correct preparation of the unit, followed by removal and disposal of all infection control barriers.

- Demonstrate appropriate image retrieval methods utilizing infection control protocol.

Introduction

The areas associated with the radiology treatment rooms are not routinely associated with the spatter of blood, body fluids, or saliva. However, radiographic procedures may pose a threat with contamination if the equipment, receptors, or treatment areas are not kept clean and sterile. The goal of this laboratory exercise is to review infection control procedures used for all patients during and after x-ray exposures.

During the x-ray exposures of patients, try to minimize contamination of surfaces by only touching the necessary equipment. Try not to handle the dental chair or controls of the chair once your gloves are contaminated. Have all supplies out and ready on the portable tray or work area to avoid the need to enter any drawer space once your gloves are contaminated. Do not touch areas of the x-ray machine that may be unwrapped, such as a section of the extension arm. If the lead apron has slipped or the thyroid collar needs adjusting, remove your gloves, wash hands, and make the correction with clean hands. After each exposure, dry the receptor and drop it in a plastic cup for completed exposures. Individual barrier pouches or envelopes should be used to reduce the risk of contamination of surfaces when the receptor is being transported and processed. Transport exposed receptors in an aseptic manner to prevent cross-contamination at the darkroom or image retrieval area.

Equipment Needed

- DXTTR teaching manikin

- infection control supplies

- x-ray film

- intraoral digital sensor

Procedure

1. Set up DXTTR, utilizing the lead apron and thyroid collar.

2. Wash hands and don gloves.

3. Turn on the x-ray machine and set the exposure control panel to the appropriate setting.

4. Prepare the radiology cubicle with appropriate infection control protocol. Assemble all prepared supplies necessary for x-ray exposure for the teaching manikin on the portable tray or covered work surface outside the cubicle.

5. Place two receptors into the plastic cup, supposing that the receptors have been exposed to radiation and are contaminated.

6. Remove gloves and wash hands. Remove lead apron from the patient as you leave the room for image retrieval.

   If using film, complete steps 7 to 12. If using digital sensors, skip to step 13.

7. Go to the darkroom with the cup of exposed films, a second empty cup for waste materials, a clean pair of gloves, and several paper towels. Place a paper towel on the work surface and place the cup with contaminated receptors next to the towel. Put on the gloves. Take one contaminated film from the cup, dry it with a paper towel, tear open the barrier envelope, and allow the film to drop onto the paper towel. Place the empty barrier envelope into the waste cup. The barriers should be discarded as infectious waste.

8. Take the second contaminated film from the cup, tear open the barrier envelope, and allow the film to drop onto the paper towel. Place the barrier envelope into the waste cup. Remove gloves and place them into the waste cup, wash hands.

9. Turn off the overhead light, turn on the safelight, and secure the darkroom door. Unwrap and process the films with clean hands.

10. If using film and a daylight loader device, place the cup of contaminated films, a second paper cup, several paper towels, and a pair of gloves into the outer compartment. Push your hands through the cuffs of the daylight loader. Place gloves on inside the compartment. Take one contaminated film from the cup, dry it with a paper towel, tear open the barrier envelope, and allow the film to drop onto the clean paper towel. Place the empty barrier envelope into the waste cup.

11. Take the second contaminated film from the cup, tear open the barrier envelope, and allow the film to drop onto the paper towel. Place the barrier envelope into the waste cup. Remove gloves and place them into the waste cup.

12. While your hands are still within the daylight loader, unwrap each film and place in the processor. Remove hands after the last film has entered the processor.

13. Handle the contaminated sensor and barrier envelope in the same manner as traditional film. Bring a second empty cup for waste materials, a clean pair of gloves, and several paper towels. Place a paper towel on the work surface and place the cup with contaminated receptors next to the towel. Put on the gloves. Allow the unwrapped sensor to be dropped onto a paper towel or into the black transfer box for scanning. Some digital manufacturers may recommend an intermediate-level disinfecting solution to wipe the surface of the sensor before scanning. After all sensors have been unwrapped, remove gloves, wash hands, and transfer the sensors in a darkened box to the scanning area. The barriers should be discarded as infectious waste.

14. Wash hands.

15. Place the teaching manikin in its storage location.

16. Place gloves on and remove all contaminated items and disposable materials and place into an appropriate area. Place the contaminated beam alignment devices into an area designated for instruments requiring sterilization.

17. With traditional radiography procedures, the lead foil should be separated from the film packet and stored for collection. Manufacturers of traditional film may offer a lead foil recycling service and should be consulted.

18. Remove barrier protection from computer keyboard and mouse, if using digital equipment. Wipe down computer equipment following manufacturer's recommendations.

19. Clean and disinfect all contaminated surfaces with the disinfecting solutions.

20. Once all waste is disposed of and equipment is clean, remove gloves and wash hands.

21. Properly store the tubehead against the wall and, if appropriate, turn off the machine and overhead lights.

CLINICAL LABORATORY ACTIVITY 3-2 WORKSHEET

Upon completion of image retrieval and infection control after exposures, ask your instructor to check that all procedures have been accomplished correctly.

PROCEDURE STEP	COMPLETED (✓)	STUDENT COMMENTS
1. Position DXTTR.		
2. Wash hands and don gloves.		
3. Turn on x-ray machine and set control panel.		
4. Assemble supplies on the portable tray or covered work surface outside the cubicle.		
5. Place exposed receptors in cup.		
6. Remove gloves and wash hands. Remove lead apron from the patient as you leave the room for image retrieval.		
7–12. Develop film.		
13. Process digital sensor.		
14. Wash hands.		
15. Remove the lead apron with clean hands and hang it in the appropriate area.		
16. Store DXTTR.		
17. Don gloves and place contaminated items in appropriate areas.		
18. Separate lead foil.		
19–20. Perform infection control procedures on equipment.		
21. Wash hands.		
22. Store tubehead.		

Faculty Signature: _____   **Date:** _____

365

4 Quality Assurance

QUALITY ASSURANCE PROCEDURES

A quality assurance plan ensures the production of high-quality images and includes both quality control tests and quality administration procedures. Quality control tests are tests that are used to monitor dental x-ray equipment, supplies, and film processing. Records of the quality assurance procedures should be kept in a notebook in the radiology clinic. The following quality control tests are recommended:

- *X-ray machine:* Dental x-ray machines should be tested for minor malfunctions, output variations, collimation problems, tubehead drift, timing errors, and inaccurate kilovoltage and milliamperage readings. These tests should be performed annually.

- *X-ray film* (Fig. 4-1): Unexposed film is available from a central dispensing area. Always check the expiration date when a new box of film is opened. If fog or other artifacts are seen on the processed film image, a fresh film test can be run to determine whether dental x-ray film is fresh and has been properly stored and protected. A fresh film test should be performed with each new box of film.

- *Screens and cassettes* (Fig. 4-2): Cassettes should be examined monthly for adequate closure, light leaks, and warping. The film-screen contact test can be used to determine the adequacy of screen-film contact. This test should be performed periodically. More frequent testing is required if the screens and cassettes are used often.

- *Digital sensors* (Fig. 4-3): Photo-stimulable phosphor (PSP) digital sensors should be periodically examined for scratches, bending, or other artifacts that may cause undiagnostic images. Direct digital sensors should be periodically examined to ensure that the wire has a tight attachment to the back of the sensor. Performance testing of digital radiography equipment must be done in accordance with manufacturer specifications.

- *Darkroom lighting:* The light leak test can be used to evaluate the darkroom for light leaks monthly. The safelighting test (Fig. 4-4) can be used to check for proper safelighting conditions and should be performed every 6 months.

- *Processing equipment and solutions:* Automatic processing equipment (Fig. 4-5) must be carefully maintained and monitored daily for potential problems. Cleaning films may be run at the beginning of the day. The level of the water bath, developer, and fixer solutions must be checked. The developer strength can be monitored by a reference radiograph or stepwedge radiograph, usually exposed on a radiography teaching manikin. The fixer solution can be checked by performing a clearing test. These tests must be performed daily. Chemicals will be replenished and processing equipment will be cleaned by designated staff members.

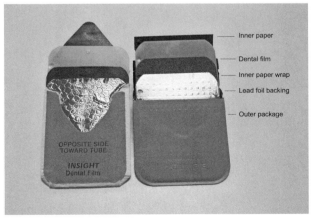

Fig. 4-1. X-ray film. Courtesy of Carestream Health Inc., Rochester, NY.

- *Miscellaneous:* Depending on your institution, additional computer equipment may be used with digital imaging. The manufacturer's recommendations should be followed for all computer updates, software downloads, and storage of image files.

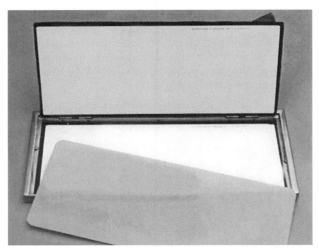

Fig. 4-2. Cassette. From White SC, Pharoah MJ: *Oral radiology: principles and interpretation*, ed 7, St. Louis: 2014, Mosby.

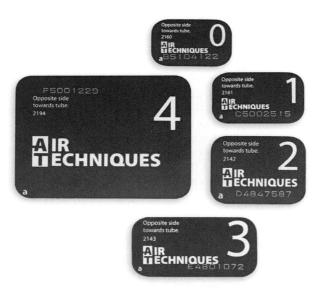

Fig. 4-3. Digital sensor. Courtesy of Air Techniques, Melville, NY.

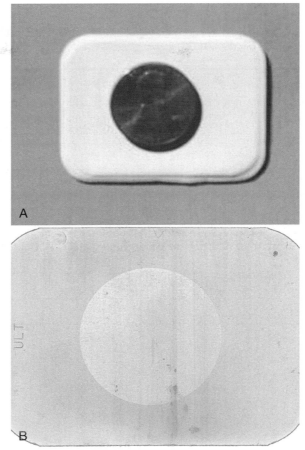

Fig. 4-4. Coin test. From Bird DL, Robinson DS: *Modern dental assisting,* ed 10, St. Louis, 2012, Saunders.

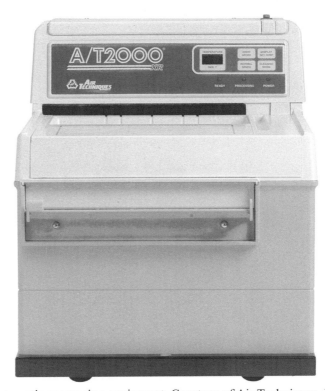

Fig. 4-5. Automatic processing equipment. Courtesy of Air Techniques, Melville, NY.

Name _____

Date _____

ASSESSMENT 4-1

Quality Assurance

1. Where is the location of documentation for quality assurance and safety for equipment used in the radiology clinic in your institution? Who performs the inspection of this equipment?

    _____

    _____

    _____

2. Who is responsible for the quality assurance procedures for equipment used in the radiology clinic, including film, sensors, processing solutions, screens and cassettes, and darkroom maintenance?

    _____

    _____

    _____

CLINIC LABORATORY ACTIVITY 4-1

Quality Assurance Tests

Objectives

- List quality control tests and quality administration procedures that should be included in the quality control plan of the institution.

- Discuss the purpose and importance of periodic testing of dental x-ray equipment.

- Describe the protocol for the following quality assurance tests: dental x-ray machines, fresh film, screens and cassettes, darkroom lighting, processing equipment and solutions, and digital imaging equipment.

Introduction

To produce diagnostic quality images, dental x-ray equipment and supplies must function properly, be kept in good repair, and be replaced if necessary. The purpose of this laboratory activity is to familiarize the student with common quality assurance tests for both traditional and digital imaging procedures.

Faculty will discuss quality control tests and administration procedures that are important to the institution. Documentation of such procedures should be presented, accompanied by certification from state or federal agencies. Students should familiarize themselves with the location and importance of such documentation.

Equipment

- newly opened box of dental x-ray film

- extraoral cassette

- stepwedge

- coin

- intraoral digital sensors

- darkroom with fresh processing chemicals, functioning safelight

Procedure

1. Faculty will demonstrate how to conduct a fresh film test, along with examples of processed fresh films and film fog.

2. Faculty will demonstrate the correct way to examine the extraoral screens and cassettes.

3. With several students at a time, faculty will demonstrate the protocol for conducting a check of the darkroom lighting and coin test for safelight effectiveness.

4. With several students at a time, faculty will demonstrate the protocol for preparing a reference or stepwedge radiograph inside the darkroom. Examples of radiographs with varying densities should be presented.

5. Faculty will demonstrate the examination of digital sensors, including the general wear and tear of sensor surfaces and wired connections.

Name _____

Date _____

TEST	STEPS	COMPLETE (✓)	RESULTS AND COMMENTS
Fresh Film Test	1. *Prepare the film.* Unwrap one unexposed film from a newly opened box.		
	2. *Process the film.* Use fresh chemicals to process the unexposed film.		
	3. *Evaluate. Film should appear clear with slight blue tint.*		
Screen-Film Contact Test	1. *Load the cassette.* Insert one film between the screens in the cassette holder and close.		
	2. *Place test object.* Place a wire mesh test object on top of the loaded cassette.		
	3. *Position the position indicating device (PID).* Position the PID using a 40-inch target-receptor distance while directing the central ray perpendicular to the cassette.		
	4. *Expose the cassette.* Expose the cassette using 10 mA, 70 kV, and 0.25 seconds.		
	5. *Process the film.* Process the exposed film.		
	6. *View.* Check the film on a view box in a dimly lit room at a distance of 6 feet.		
	7. *Evaluate.* Adequate contact has uniform density.		
Safelighting Test (Coin Test)	1. *Prepare the darkroom.* Turn off all the lights in the darkroom, including the safelight.		
	2. *Prepare the film.* Unwrap one unexposed film. Place it on a flat surface at least 4 feet from the safelight. Place a coin on top of the film.		
	3. *Turn on the safelight.* Allow the film and the coin to be exposed to the safelight for 3 to 4 minutes.		
	4. *Process the film.* Remove the coin and process the film.		
	5. *Evaluate.* Outline of coin should not appear.		
Reference Radiograph	1. *Prepare the film.* Use fresh film to make a reference radiograph. Place an aluminum stepwedge on top of the film.		
	2. *Expose the film,* using correct exposure factors. With Insight film, use 65 kV, 7 mA, and an exposure time of 0.13 to 0.14 seconds.		
	3. *Process the film* using fresh chemicals at the recommended time and temperature.		

TEST	STEPS	COMPLETE (✓)	RESULTS AND COMMENTS
Stepwedge-Radiograph	1. *Prepare the films.* Use a total of 20 fresh films to create a 1-month supply of films for daily testing. Place an aluminum stepwedge on top of one film.		
	2. *Expose the film.* Repeat with the remaining films using the same stepwedge, same target-receptor distance, and same exposure factors. With INSIGHT film, use 65 kV, 7 mA, and an exposure time of 0.13 to 0.14 seconds.		
	3. Using fresh chemicals, process only one of the exposed films. This processed radiograph is known as the standard stepwedge radiograph.		
	4. Store the remaining 19 exposed films in a cool, dry area protected from x-radiation.		
	5. Each day, after the chemicals have been replenished, process <u>one</u> of the exposed stepwedge films. This film is known as the daily radiograph.		
	6. *View the standard radiograph and the daily radiograph side by side on a view box.* Compare the densities seen on the daily radiograph with the densities seen on the standard radiograph.		
Digital sensor examination	1. Examine digital sensors, including the general wear and tear of sensor surfaces and wired connections.		

Faculty Signature: _____   **Date:** _____

The dental radiographer must have a working knowledge of techniques used for acquiring intraoral and extraoral images. The majority of this portion of the laboratory manual is concentrated on learning these techniques with the goal of producing diagnostic images.

ORDER OF THE LABORATORY EXERCISES

DXTTR Exercises
- Bisecting technique: anterior, posterior periapical images
- Bite-wing technique: with tabs
- **Bisecting Technique Competency Exam: ½ of a full mouth series**
- Paralleling technique: anterior, posterior periapical images
- Bite-wing technique: with beam alignment devices
- **Paralleling Technique Competency Exam: ½ of a full mouth series**
- Occlusal technique: maxillary and mandibular occlusal images

Peer Patient Exercises (NO exposures will be made on students)
- Bisecting technique: anterior, posterior periapical images
- Bite-wing technique: with tabs
- Paralleling technique: anterior, posterior periapical images
- Bite-wing technique: with beam alignment devices
- Occlusal technique: maxillary and mandibular occlusal images
- Panoramic technique: demonstration and peer patient exercise
- **Paralleling Technique Competency Exam: full mouth series (no exposures)**
- **Panoramic Technique Competency Exam (no exposures)**

By the end of these laboratory sessions, students will have the opportunity to learn the following techniques: bisecting, paralleling, bite-wing, occlusal and panoramic. Depending on school policy, a level of competency in each area must be achieved before proceeding with the next technique. Competency examinations will be administered to evaluate student progress and ensure that students not only understand the techniques but also can produce diagnostic images.

Competency Exams

Two competency exams will be administered with the teaching manikin. For these two exams, students will be required to expose ½ of a complete mouth series (approximately ten images) in a timed setting. Thirty minutes is a suggested time limit for these exams, not including the time needed for image retrieval.

- The *Bisecting Technique Competency Exam* includes two maxillary anterior images, two mandibular anterior images, two maxillary posterior images, two mandibular posterior images, and two bite-wing images exposed on the RIGHT side of DXTTR.
- The *Paralleling Technique Competency Exam* includes two maxillary anterior images, two mandibular anterior images, two maxillary posterior images, two mandibular posterior images, and two bite-wing images exposed on the LEFT side of DXTTR.

The third competency exam will be administered with peer patients. Students will be divided into pairs and will be required to "expose" a complete mouth series (approximately 18 images) in a timed setting on their partner. No student will be exposed to radiation! Forty-five minutes is a suggested time limit for this exam.

- *Paralleling Technique Exam* on a Peer Patient includes three (or more) maxillary anterior image placements, three mandibular anterior image placements, four maxillary posterior image placements, four mandibular posterior image placements, and four bite-wing image placements.

Faculty will grade the peer patient competency exam on lead apron placement, receptor placement, exposure sequence, infection control, PID alignment, correct assembly of beam alignment devices and patient management. Since no student is exposed to radiation, no images will be produced. Therefore, it is critical that faculty observe the students very closely during the complete mouth series.

The fourth and final competency exam will be given after students receive a demonstration on the operations of the panoramic machine and correct exposure technique (Figure 5-1). Once the presentation is complete, students may be placed in groups of three: one student will act as the patient, one will act as the operator, and one will act as the fac-ulty member. It will be the responsibility of the "faculty member" to evaluate proper positioning, patient management.

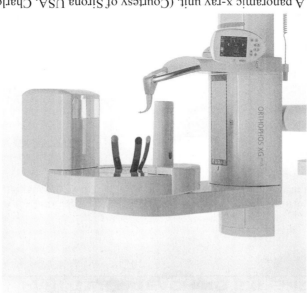

Fig. 5-1. A panoramic x-ray unit. (Courtesy of Sirona USA, Charlotte, NC)

infection control procedures, and appropriate instructions given to the "patient." Students will then rotate, allowing everyone an opportunity to function in one of these three roles.

Bisecting vs. Paralleling

Although the paralleling technique is listed first in the textbook under "Technique Basics," it is the suggestion of the author to teach the bisecting technique prior to the paralleling technique. The bisecting technique is typically a more difficult intraoral technique to master because the student is responsible for the correct vertical and horizontal angulation, as well as the precise alignment of the PID with the intraoral receptor.

The bisecting technique (along with learning to expose bite-wing images with tabs) requires the students to understand the rule of isometry, seeing the results of choosing too much or too little vertical angulation. The bisecting technique teaches students how to select the correct horizontal angulation and visualize the central ray opening up the interproximal contact areas. The bisecting technique challenges students to imagine the dimensions and position of the intraoral receptor in aligning the PID to completely cover the surface area of the receptor before exposure.

It is a great achievement to overcome the disadvantages of the bisecting technique and produce diagnostic images. Once this first hurdle is completed, the paralleling technique will appear more manageable and simpler. Students typically do extremely well mastering the paralleling technique after the laborious bisecting technique. However, it is the discretion of the faculty to decide the order of the laboratory exercises.

PRESCRIBED PLACEMENTS FOR INTRAORAL RECEPTORS

Suggested receptor placements for all intraoral exposures are designed to give the most diagnostic information possible of the maxillary and mandibular arches. These guidelines illustrate which teeth and surrounding anatomy should be visible on each image. Descriptions of the prescribed placements and radiographic examples will follow in the laboratory manual.

Due to the various sizes and thicknesses of some sensors, it may be difficult to capture all of the structures recommended. Faculty should decide which images are diagnostic and which did not adequately cover the area of interest.

- For example, if mandibular third molars are present and horizontally-oriented, the molar periapical image that includes the distal of the second premolar may not capture the apices of the mandibular third molar. This situation may be considered an error in packet placement when in fact the scenario may warrant the need of a panoramic image.

- Another situation is the patient who requires premolar bite-wing images but presents with a small mouth and limited opening, or mandibular lingual tori. A digital sensor may not be positioned far enough forward to include the distal of the mandibular canine due to the bulk or size of the receptor. Most dentists would prefer open interproximal contact areas of the premolar teeth rather than severe overlap with the distal of the canine present.

The maxillary anterior region seems to generate much variation in the number and size of receptors needed to adequately image this area. Some institutions may require anywhere from six to ten images; the author recommends the minimal number of images while still providing enough diagnostic information to properly evaluate the twelve teeth of the anterior maxilla.

EXPOSURE SEQUENCE

Exposure sequences are recommended for each technique. Step-by-step exposure sequences are specified to ensure that all students are following the same criteria. Please note that several digital imaging manufacturers have integrated an exposure sequence into their software. Step-by-step exposure sequences are specified to ensure that all students are following the same criteria. Please note that several digital imaging manufacturers have integrated an exposure sequence into their software; the operator cannot choose the order of exposures. However, an established exposure sequence is recommended for each intraoral technique in this laboratory manual, to prevent errors, to encourage students to follow an exposure routine, and to use time efficiently.

GRADING OF IMAGES

The laboratory sessions that include graded assignments should be evaluated in the same manner as the grading of the competency examinations. Remember that errors can occur during radiographic exposures as well as during image retrieval procedures, such as in the darkroom or with computer software. Mounting images correctly is also a part of the laboratory sessions and competency exams. A suggested grading scale for images is as follows:

- Each image has the potential for earning five points. An image that is positioned, exposed and retrieved correctly with no errors earns a score of five points.
- Small or minor errors that do not overly affect the diagnostic quality of the image, such as a slight cone-cut (Figure 5-2), may result in a one-point deduction. An image may also display several minor errors (slight horizontal angulation, slight receptor placement) and one point should be deducted for each error present.
- A major error, such as a large cone-cut, a backwards film (Figure 5-3), or a totally black image earns a score of zero points for that image.
- Failure of the laboratory exercise may occur if the student does not utilize the lead apron prior to exposures, or for any major violations of infection control protocol. Failure may also occur if the images are incorrectly mounted. This decision will be at the discretion of the faculty.

If the laboratory exercise requires four bite-wing images, a total of twenty points is possible for that assignment (four images at five points each). A perfect bite-wing exercise would produce 20/20 points, or 100%.

If a complete mouth series of images (total of 18) were exposed on DXTTR, the student would have the opportunity to score a possibility of 90 points (18 images @ five points each). Again, points would be deducted for minor and major errors, image retrieval, or mounting issues.

Each institution has guidelines stating the grades required to reach competency. The faculty will decide what grade is considered to be "passing" for the laboratory exercises and competency examinations. For example, a minimum grade of 75% may be required to pass the radiology course.

INTRODUCTION TO THE LABORATORY EXERCISES

As mentioned in the equipment section, the teaching manikin used in the radiographic technique exercises is DXTTR (Fig. 5-4). Please handle the manikin *carefully* and ensure that it is firmly attached to the dental chair (or other working surface) before beginning any assignments. Inform a faculty or staff member if difficulties arise with the proper function-ing of the manikin. Proper storage and handling is also important. Please handle with extreme care!

After the intraoral techniques and competency examinations have been completed, students will have the opportunity to perform these skills on each other, referred to as "peer patient exercises." These exercises allow students not only to act as the dental radiographer but, equally important, to sit as the dental patient and undergo the radiology experience firsthand.

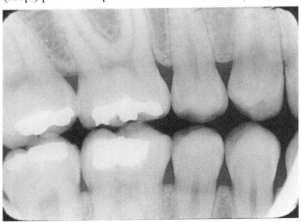

Fig. 5-2. A cone-cut is an example of a minor error, seen as a curved unexposed (clear) area on the image.

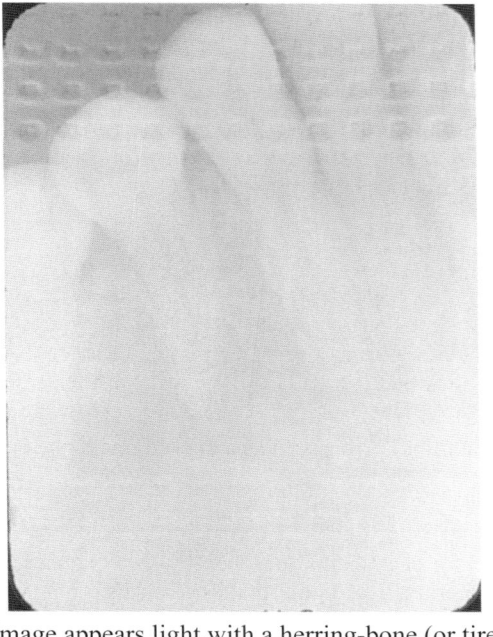

Fig. 5-3. If the film is reversed, the image appears light with a herring-bone (or tire-track) pattern. This is an example of a major error.

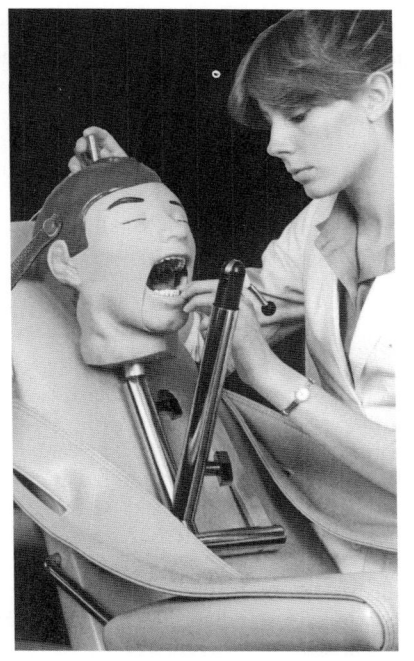

Fig. 5-4. DXTTR training manikin. Courtesy of Dentsply Rinn, York, PA.

Peer patient exercises allow students time to strengthen the techniques learned through the teaching manikin and also reinforce patient management skills. We suggest students rotate through the peer patient exercises and change partners as frequently as possible, time permitting. This will give the student many opportunities with various patient anatomic conditions.

Although infection control procedures have been suggested for use up to this point, adhering to standard precautions plays a very important role in the peer patient exercises. Students can appreciate immediately the significance of infection control procedures used in film-based and digital imaging systems in the preparation of units, exposure, and image retrieval phases of radiography.

378

As students prepare for peer patient exercises, it is important to remember that *no exposures will be made on fellow classmates*. This technique section concentrates on intraoral technique, patient management, and infection control procedures. Faculty and staff members will critique student performance based on obvious errors that may be seen, *without exposures*.

The final section of the technique portion of this manual concentrates on panoramic radiography. Panoramic imaging is one of the most common forms of extraoral images and is typically found in most dental offices. The panoramic image allows the dental professional to view larger areas of the maxilla and mandible in comparison to the periapical, bite-wing, or occlusal views.

For a panoramic image to be diagnostic, correct patient positioning and preparation is critical. The student must be familiar with the panoramic machine, focal trough, head positioning tools, exposure controls, and the cassette that encases the receptor. Although the use of extraoral machines varies by manufacturer, general guidelines are presented that should be applicable to many panoramic units.

Please leave the radiology cubicle and surrounding areas clean and stocked with supplies at the end of each laboratory exercise. Even if the previous operator did not clean the area well, everyone else will appreciate your extra steps to clean, disinfect, and restock all supplies, and leave the x-ray machine firmly against the wall. *Thank you!*

5 | Bisecting Technique

BASIC CONCEPTS OF THE BISECTING TECHNIQUE

- Place the receptor along the lingual surface of the teeth.

- The long axis of the tooth and plane of the receptor form an angle at the point where the receptor contacts the tooth.

- Visualize a plane that divides in half the angle formed by the long axis of the tooth and the receptor; this plane is termed the "imaginary bisector."

- Direct the central ray perpendicular to the imaginary bisector.

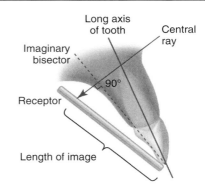

CLINICAL LABORATORY ACTIVITY 5.1

Bisecting Technique: Anterior Periapical Images

Objectives

- Discuss the rule of isometry and how it pertains to this intraoral technique.

- Illustrate the location of the receptor, tooth, imaginary bisector, and central ray.

- Describe the receptor size(s) used with the bisecting technique in the anterior region.

- Describe correct and incorrect horizontal and vertical angulation.

- Explain the correct sequence of exposure of the anterior projections.

- Discuss the advantages and disadvantages of the bisecting technique.

Introduction

The goal of this laboratory exercise is to use the training manikin to produce diagnostic images of the maxillary and mandibular anterior teeth utilizing the bisecting technique. Depending on school policy, between six and eight total projections are exposed to cover the following areas: maxillary right and left canine, maxillary incisors, mandibular right and left canine, and mandibular incisors.

EXAMPLES OF MOUNTED DIAGNOSTIC ANTERIOR PERIAPICAL IMAGES

Maxillary Canine

- The entire crown and root of the canine, including the apex and the surrounding structures, must be seen on this image.

- The interproximal alveolar bone and mesial contact of the canine must also be visible.

- The lingual cusp of the first premolar usually obscures the distal contact of the canine.

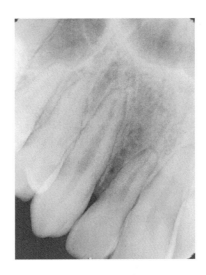

Maxillary Incisor

- The entire crowns and roots of all four maxillary incisors, including the apices of the teeth and the surrounding structures, must be seen on this image.

- The interproximal alveolar bone between the central incisors and the central and lateral incisors must also be visible.

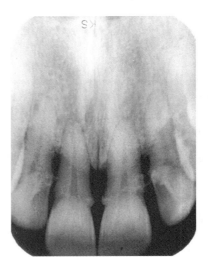

Mandibular Canine

- The entire crown and root of the canine, including the apex and the surrounding structures, must be seen on this image.

- The interproximal alveolar bone and mesial and distal contacts must also be visible.

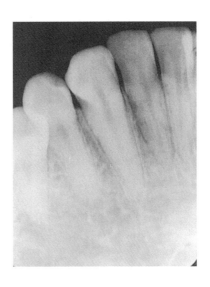

Mandibular Incisor

- The entirety of the crowns and roots of the four mandibular incisors, including the apices of the teeth and the surrounding structures, must be seen on this image.

- The contacts between the central incisors and between the central and lateral incisors must also be visible.

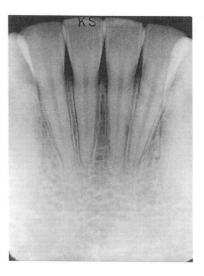

Exposure Sequence

Use the following exposure sequence for the anterior periapical images:

1. maxillary right canine

2. maxillary incisors

3. maxillary left canine

4. mandibular left canine

5. mandibular incisors

6. mandibular right canine

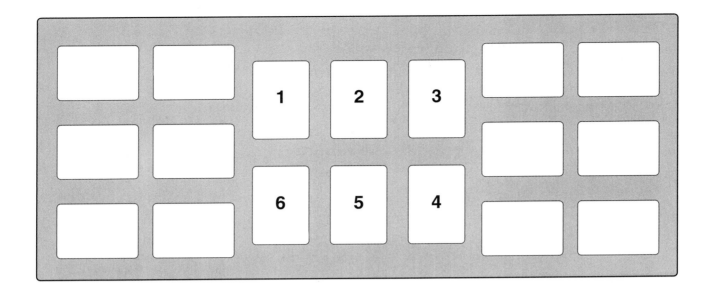

Equipment Needed

- radiology cubicle prepared with appropriate infection control protocol

- training manikin

- lead apron and thyroid collar

- receptors for anterior projections (size 1 and/or 2 depending on your institution) in a plastic cup

- disposable bite blocks

- cotton rolls

Procedure

1. Set up DXTTR, utilizing the lead apron and thyroid collar.

2. Wash hands and don gloves.

3. Place receptors, cup, bite blocks, and cotton rolls on the covered work surface in a radiation-safe area, just outside the radiology cubicle.

4. Turn on the x-ray machine and set the exposure control panel to the appropriate setting for the maxillary canine projection.

5. Enter the radiology cubicle and move the tubehead into the area near the maxillary right canine.

6. Picture the placement of the receptor inside the mouth, and try to visualize the imaginary angle created between the receptor and the tooth. Align the position indicating device (PID) to bisect the imaginary line created between the receptor and tooth. The central ray of radiation should be directed at a 90-degree angle to the imaginary bisector.

7. Also, try to visualize the central ray directed through the teeth, opening up the contact areas. Place the PID as close to these correct settings as possible *before* the receptor is inside the mouth.

8. Over the covered work surface, place the first receptor in a vertical direction snugly into the bite block.

9. Re-enter the cubicle and place the receptor and bite block into the mouth of the teaching manikin, centered on tooth #6. Close training manikin carefully on the bite block.

10. Recheck your vertical and horizontal angulations. Cover the entire receptor with the outline of the PID.

11. Expose the periapical image.

12. Place the exposed receptor into a clean disposable cup in a radiation-safe area.

13. Continue to make exposures in the maxillary anterior region. Follow the exposure sequence listed previously. When the maxillary anterior teeth are complete, adjust the control panel if necessary for mandibular anterior exposures.

14. When all exposures are complete, remove gloves, wash hands, and remove the lead apron and thyroid collar. Proceed to the darkroom or image retrieval area to process the radiographs.

15. Once all images have been retrieved, place in anatomic order with either a film mount or computer software. Evaluate your anterior exposures with the use of the image critique form that follows this Laboratory Activity. Note that only the anterior exposures should be evaluated at this time. When images are mounted and critiqued, inform the faculty and receive feedback.

Image Critique Form

Students: Evaluate the images created for this lab session. Use the letters in the Critique Key to describe errors seen on the images. Label each exposure with any errors seen.

Student Name: _____   Patient Name: _____   Date of Exam: _____   Grade: _____

Area Exposed	Student Evaluation of Error	Retakes* (Y)	Pt Management Issues* (need faculty signature)	Faculty Evaluation of Error*
Max Right Molar				
Max Right Premolar				
Max Right Canine				
Max Centrals				
Max Left Canine				
Max Left Premolar				
Max Left Molar				
Right Molar Bite-wing				
Right Premolar Bite-wing				
Left Premolar Bite-wing				
Left Molar Bite-wing				
Mand Right Molar				
Mand Right Premolar				
Mand Right Canine				
Mand Centrals				
Mand Left Canine				
Mand Left Premolar				
Mand Left Molar				
PANORAMIC RADIOGRAPH				

Critique Key

B = exposed backwards
C = cone-cut
E = elongation
F = foreshortening
FM = mounting error
H = horizontal angulation
IC = infection control error
LA = failure to place lead apron
M = movement
Ms = misc (specify)
P = receptor placement
PR = processing (specify)
R = retake (specify)
FP = Frankfort plane (up/down)
FT = focal trough (ant/post)
G = ghost image
MID = midsagittal plane
LAA = lead apron artifact

*Faculty: Review the images and critique as necessary; decide if retakes are necessary. Patient management issues may be documented in future semesters.

Module **5** Bisecting Technique

Image Critique Form

Students: Evaluate the images created for this lab session. Use the letters in the Critique Key to describe errors seen on the images. Label each exposure with any errors seen.

Student Name: _____   Patient Name: _____   Date of Exam: _____   Grade: _____

Area Exposed	Student Evaluation of Error	Retakes* (Y)	Pt Management Issues* (need faculty signature)	Faculty Evaluation of Error*
Max Right Molar				
Max Right Premolar				
Max Right Canine				
Max Centrals				
Max Left Canine				
Max Left Premolar				
Max Left Molar				
Right Molar Bite-wing				
Right Premolar Bite-wing				
Left Premolar Bite-wing				
Left Molar Bite-wing				
Mand Right Molar				
Mand Right Premolar				
Mand Right Canine				
Mand Centrals				
Mand Left Canine				
Mand Left Premolar				
Mand Left Molar				
PANORAMIC RADIOGRAPH				

Critique Key

B = exposed backwards
C = cone-cut
E = elongation
F = foreshortening
FM = mounting error
H = horizontal angulation
IC = infection control error
LA = failure to place lead apron
M = movement
Ms = misc (specify)
P = receptor placement
PR = processing (specify)
R = retake (specify)
FP = Frankfort plane (up/down)
FT = focal trough (ant/post)
G = ghost image
MID = midsagittal plane
LAA = lead apron artifact

*Faculty: Review the images and critique as necessary; decide if retakes are necessary. Patient management issues may be documented in future semesters.

Image Critique Form

Students: Evaluate the images created for this lab session. Use the letters in the Critique Key to describe errors seen on the images. Label each exposure with any errors seen.

Student Name: _____ Patient Name: _____ Date of Exam: _____ Grade: _____

Area Exposed	Student Evaluation of Error	Retakes* (Y)	Pt Management Issues* (need faculty signature)	Faculty Evaluation of Error*
Max Right Molar				
Max Right Premolar				
Max Right Canine				
Max Centrals				
Max Left Canine				
Max Left Premolar				
Max Left Molar				
Right Molar Bite-wing				
Right Premolar Bite-wing				
Left Premolar Bite-wing				
Left Molar Bite-wing				
Mand Right Molar				
Mand Right Premolar				
Mand Right Canine				
Mand Centrals				
Mand Left Canine				
Mand Left Premolar				
Mand Left Molar				
PANORAMIC RADIOGRAPH				

Critique Key

B = exposed backwards
C = cone-cut
E = elongation
F = foreshortening
FM = mounting error
H = horizontal angulation
IC = infection control error
LA = failure to place lead apron
M = movement
Ms = misc (specify)
P = receptor placement
PR = processing (specify)
R = retake (specify)
FP = Frankfort plane (up/down)
FT = focal trough (ant/post)
G = ghost image
MID = midsagittal plane
LAA = lead apron artifact

*Faculty: Review the images and critique as necessary; decide if retakes are necessary. Patient management issues may be documented in future semesters.

Image Critique Form

Students: Evaluate the images created for this lab session. Use the letters in the Critique Key to describe errors seen on the images. Label each exposure with any errors seen.

Student Name: _____ Patient Name: _____ Date of Exam: _____ Grade: _____

Area Exposed	Student Evaluation of Error	Retakes* (Y)	Pt Management Issues* (need faculty signature)	Faculty Evaluation of Error*
Max Right Molar				
Max Right Premolar				
Max Right Canine				
Max Centrals				
Max Left Canine				
Max Left Premolar				
Max Left Molar				
Right Molar Bite-wing				
Right Premolar Bite-wing				
Left Premolar Bite-wing				
Left Molar Bite-wing				
Mand Right Molar				
Mand Right Premolar				
Mand Right Canine				
Mand Centrals				
Mand Left Canine				
Mand Left Premolar				
Mand Left Molar				
PANORAMIC RADIOGRAPH				

Critique Key

B = exposed backwards
C = cone-cut
E = elongation
F = foreshortening
FM = mounting error
H = horizontal angulation
IC = infection control error
LA = failure to place lead apron
M = movement
Ms = misc (specify)
P = receptor placement
PR = processing (specify)
R = retake (specify)
FP = Frankfort plane (up/down)
FT = focal trough (ant/post)
G = ghost image
MID = midsagittal plane
LAA = lead apron artifact

*Faculty: Review the images and critique as necessary; decide if retakes are necessary. Patient management issues may be documented in future semesters.

CLINICAL LABORATORY ACTIVITY 5-1 WORKSHEET

Questions for Group Discussion

1. In what situations would the bisecting technique be preferred over the paralleling technique?

_____

_____

_____

2. What factors determine the horizontal and vertical angulations chosen for each projection?

_____

_____

_____

3. What was easy about using this intraoral radiographic technique? Why?

_____

_____

_____

4. What was difficult about using this intraoral radiographic technique? Why?

_____

_____

_____

5. Years ago, this technique was accomplished with the use of the patient's finger holding the receptor in place. Why is this technique not recommended today?

_____

_____

_____

Objectives

- Describe the receptor size(s) used with the bisecting technique in the posterior region.

- Describe correct and incorrect horizontal and vertical angulation.

- Describe patient and equipment preparations necessary before using the bisecting technique.

- Explain the correct sequence of exposure of the posterior projections.

Introduction

The goal of this laboratory exercise is to produce diagnostic images with the training manikin of the maxillary and mandibular posterior teeth utilizing the bisecting technique. Eight total projections must be exposed to cover the following areas: maxillary right and left premolar and molar regions, and mandibular right and left premolar and molar regions.

EXAMPLES OF MOUNTED DIAGNOSTIC POSTERIOR PERIAPICAL IMAGES

Maxillary Premolar

- All crowns and roots of the first and second premolars and first molar, including the apices, alveolar crests, contact areas, and surrounding bone, must be seen on this image.

- The distal contact of the maxillary canine must be visible in this projection.

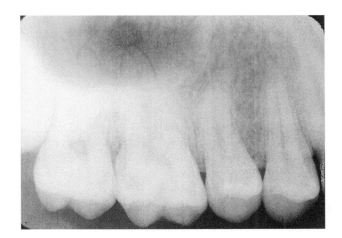

Maxillary Molar

- All crowns and roots of the first, second, and third molars, including the apices, alveolar crests, contact areas, surrounding bone, and tuberosity region, must be seen on this image.

- The distal contact of the maxillary second premolar must be visible in this projection.

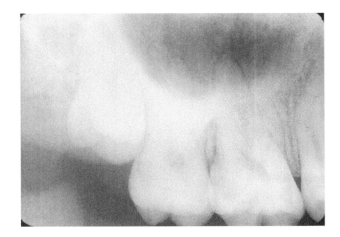

Mandibular Premolar

- All crowns and roots of the first and second premolars and first molar, including the apices, alveolar crests, contact areas, and surrounding bone, must be seen on this image.

- The distal contact of the mandibular canine should be visible in this projection.

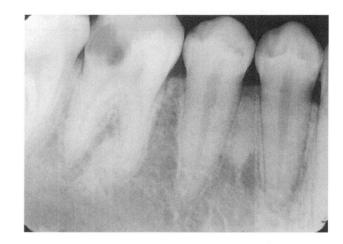

Mandibular Molar

- All crowns and roots of the first, second, and third molars, including the apices, alveolar crests, contact areas, and surrounding bone, must be seen on this image.

- The distal contact of the mandibular second premolar must be visible in this projection.

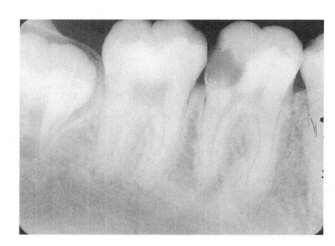

Exposure Sequence

Use the following exposure sequence for the posterior periapical images:

1. maxillary right premolar

2. maxillary right molar

3. maxillary left premolar

4. maxillary left molar

5. mandibular left premolar

6. mandibular left molar

7. mandibular right premolar

8. mandibular right molar

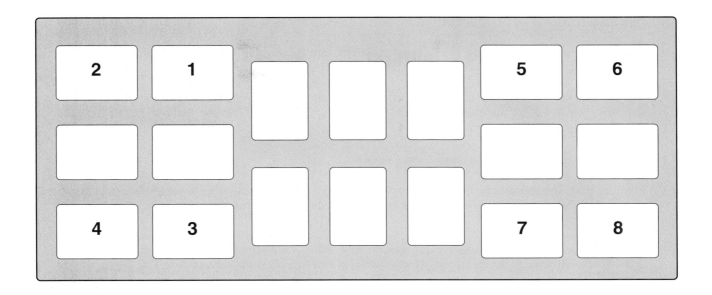

Equipment Needed

- radiology cubicle prepared with appropriate infection control protocol

- training manikin

- lead apron and thyroid collar

- receptors for posterior projections (size 1 and/or 2 depending on your institution) in a plastic cup

- disposable bite blocks

- cotton rolls

Procedure

1. Set up DXTTR, utilizing the lead apron and thyroid collar.

2. Wash hands and place gloves on.

3. Place receptors, cup, bite blocks, and cotton rolls on the covered work surface in a radiation-safe area, just outside the radiology cubicle.

4. Turn on x-ray machine and set control panel to appropriate exposure settings for the maxillary premolar projection.

5. Enter the radiology cubicle, and move the tubehead into the area near the maxillary right premolar.

6. Picture the placement of the receptor inside the mouth, and try to visualize the imaginary angle created between the receptor and the tooth. Align the PID to bisect the imaginary line created between the receptor and tooth. The central ray of radiation should be directed at a 90-degree angle to the imaginary bisector.

7. Also, try to visualize the central ray directed through the teeth, opening up the contact areas. Place the PID as close to these correct settings as possible *before* the receptor is inside the mouth.

8. Over the covered work surface, place the first receptor in a horizontal direction snugly into the bite block.

9. Reenter the cubicle and place the receptor and bite block into the mouth of the teaching manikin, centered on teeth #4 and #5. Close training manikin carefully on the bite block.

10. Recheck your vertical and horizontal angulations. Cover the entire receptor with the outline of the PID.

11. Expose the periapical image.

12. Place the exposed receptor into a clean disposable cup.

13. Continue to make exposures in the maxillary posterior region. Follow the exposure sequence listed previously. When the maxillary posterior teeth are complete, adjust the control panel if necessary for mandibular posterior exposures.

14. When all exposures are complete, remove gloves, wash hands, and remove the lead apron and thyroid collar. Proceed to the darkroom or image retrieval area to process the radiographs.

15. Once all images have been retrieved, place in anatomic order with either a film mount or computer software. Evaluate your posterior exposures with the use of the image critique form on the next page. Note that only the posterior exposures should be evaluated at this time. When images are mounted and critiqued, inform the faculty to receive feedback.

Image Critique Form

Students: Evaluate the images created for this lab session. Use the letters in the Critique Key to describe errors seen on the images. Label each exposure with any errors seen.

Student Name: _____   Patient Name: _____   Date of Exam: _____   Grade: _____

Critique Key

B = exposed backwards
C = cone-cut
E = elongation
F = foreshortening
FM = mounting error
H = horizontal angulation
IC = infection control error
LA = failure to place lead apron
M = movement
Ms = misc (specify)
P = receptor placement
PR = processing (specify)
R = retake (specify)
FP = Frankfort plane (up/down)
FT = focal trough (ant/post)
G = ghost image
MID = midsagittal plane
LAA = lead apron artifact

Area Exposed	Student Evaluation of Error	Retakes* (Y)	Pt Management Issues* (need faculty signature)	Faculty Evaluation of Error*
Max Right Molar				
Max Right Premolar				
Max Right Canine				
Max Centrals				
Max Left Canine				
Max Left Premolar				
Max Left Molar				
Right Molar Bite-wing				
Right Premolar Bite-wing				
Left Premolar Bite-wing				
Left Molar Bite-wing				
Mand Right Molar				
Mand Right Premolar				
Mand Right Canine				
Mand Centrals				
Mand Left Canine				
Mand Left Premolar				
Mand Left Molar				
PANORAMIC RADIOGRAPH				

*Faculty: Review the images and critique as necessary; decide if retakes are necessary. Patient management issues may be documented in future semesters.

Image Critique Form

Students: Evaluate the images created for this lab session. Use the letters in the Critique Key to describe errors seen on the images. Label each exposure with any errors seen.

Student Name: _____ Patient Name: _____ Date of Exam: _____ Grade: _____

Area Exposed	Student Evaluation of Error	Retakes* (Y)	Pt Management Issues* (need faculty signature)	Faculty Evaluation of Error*
Max Right Molar				
Max Right Premolar				
Max Right Canine				
Max Centrals				
Max Left Canine				
Max Left Premolar				
Max Left Molar				
Right Molar Bite-wing				
Right Premolar Bite-wing				
Left Premolar Bite-wing				
Left Molar Bite-wing				
Mand Right Molar				
Mand Right Premolar				
Mand Right Canine				
Mand Centrals				
Mand Left Canine				
Mand Left Premolar				
Mand Left Molar				
PANORAMIC RADIOGRAPH				

Critique Key

B = exposed backwards
C = cone-cut
E = elongation
F = foreshortening
FM = mounting error
H = horizontal angulation
IC = infection control error
LA = failure to place lead apron
M = movement
Ms = misc (specify)
P = receptor placement
PR = processing (specify)
R = retake (specify)
FP = Frankfort plane (up/down)
FT = focal trough (ant/post)
G = ghost image
MID = midsagittal plane
LAA = lead apron artifact

*Faculty: Review the images and critique as necessary; decide if retakes are necessary. Patient management issues may be documented in future semesters.

Image Critique Form

Students: Evaluate the images created for this lab session. Use the letters in the Critique Key to describe errors seen on the images. Label each exposure with any errors seen.

Student Name: _____   Patient Name: _____   Date of Exam: _____   Grade: _____

Critique Key

B = exposed backwards
C = cone-cut
E = elongation
F = foreshortening
FM = mounting error
H = horizontal angulation
IC = infection control error
LA = failure to place lead apron
M = movement
Ms = misc (specify)
P = receptor placement
PR = processing (specify)
R = retake (specify)
FP = Frankfort plane (up/down)
FT = focal trough (ant/post)
G = ghost image
MID = midsagittal plane
LAA = lead apron artifact

Area Exposed	Student Evaluation of Error	Retakes* (Y)	Pt Management Issues* (need faculty signature)	Faculty Evaluation of Error*
Max Right Molar				
Max Right Premolar				
Max Right Canine				
Max Centrals				
Max Left Canine				
Max Left Premolar				
Max Left Molar				
Right Molar Bite-wing				
Right Premolar Bite-wing				
Left Premolar Bite-wing				
Left Molar Bite-wing				
Mand Right Molar				
Mand Right Premolar				
Mand Right Canine				
Mand Centrals				
Mand Left Canine				
Mand Left Premolar				
Mand Left Molar				
PANORAMIC RADIOGRAPH				

*Faculty: Review the images and critique as necessary; decide if retakes are necessary. Patient management issues may be documented in future semesters.

Image Critique Form

Students: Evaluate the images created for this lab session. Use the letters in the Critique Key to describe errors seen on the images. Label each exposure with any errors seen.

Student Name: _____ Patient Name: _____ Date of Exam: _____ Grade: _____

Area Exposed	Student Evaluation of Error	Retakes* (Y)	Pt Management Issues* (need faculty signature)	Faculty Evaluation of Error*
Max Right Molar				
Max Right Premolar				
Max Right Canine				
Max Centrals				
Max Left Canine				
Max Left Premolar				
Max Left Molar				
Right Molar Bite-wing				
Right Premolar Bite-wing				
Left Premolar Bite-wing				
Left Molar Bite-wing				
Mand Right Molar				
Mand Right Premolar				
Mand Right Canine				
Mand Centrals				
Mand Left Canine				
Mand Left Premolar				
Mand Left Molar				
PANORAMIC RADIOGRAPH				

Critique Key

B = exposed backwards
C = cone-cut
E = elongation
F = foreshortening
FM = mounting error
H = horizontal angulation
IC = infection control error
LA = failure to place lead apron
M = movement
Ms = misc (specify)
P = receptor placement
PR = processing (specify)
R = retake (specify)
FP = Frankfort plane (up/down)
FT = focal trough (ant/post)
G = ghost image
MID = midsagittal plane
LAA = lead apron artifact

*Faculty: Review the images and critique as necessary; decide if retakes are necessary. Patient management issues may be documented in future semesters.

CLINICAL LABORATORY ACTIVITY 5-2 WORKSHEET

Questions for Group Discussion

1. What clinical situations may make the posterior exposures more difficult for the patient?

   _____

   _____

   _____

2. What clinical situations may make the posterior exposures more difficult for the operator?

   _____

   _____

   _____

3. Why is the premolar placement always exposed *before* the molar placement?

   _____

   _____

   _____

4. What modifications would be made with the receptor placement if the patient were missing several posterior teeth?

   _____

   _____

   _____

5. Which exposures were easier, maxillary posterior or mandibular posterior? Why?

   _____

   _____

   _____

6 Bite-Wing Technique with Tabs: Exposures, Mounting, and Critique

BASIC CONCEPTS OF THE BITE-WING TECHNIQUE

- Place the receptor in the mouth parallel to the crowns of the maxillary and mandibular posterior teeth.

- The patient bites on the tab attached to the receptor.

- The vertical angulation is set at +10 degrees; the horizontal angulation is directed through the contact areas of the posterior teeth.

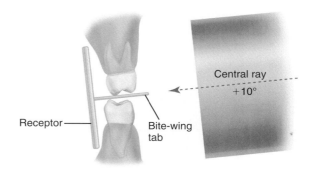

Central ray +10°

Receptor

Bite-wing tab

CLINICAL LABORATORY ACTIVITY 6-1

Bite-Wing with Tabs Technique

Objectives

- Discuss the basic principles of the bite-wing technique and illustrate the locations of the receptor, tooth, and central ray for both premolar and molar placements.

- Describe the correct vertical and horizontal angulations used with the bite-wing tab technique.

- Describe the receptor size used with the bite-wing technique.

- Describe patient and equipment preparations necessary before using the bite-wing technique.

- Explain the correct sequence of exposure of the premolar and molar projections; explain the correct sequence when the bite-wing exposures are part of a full-mouth series.

Introduction

The goal of this laboratory exercise is to use the training manikin to produce diagnostic images of the maxillary and mandibular posterior teeth utilizing the bite-wing technique with tabs (Fig. 6-1). Four total projections are exposed to cover the following areas: right and left premolar and molar regions.

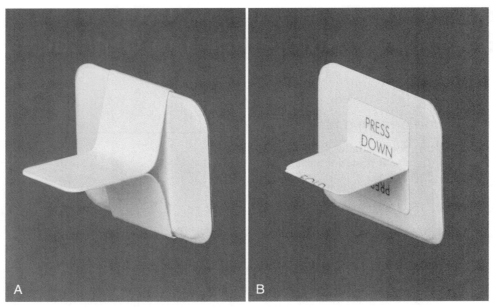

Fig. 6-1. A, Bite-wing with tabs. **B,** Adhesive bite-wing tabs.

EXAMPLES OF MOUNTED DIAGNOSTIC BITE-WING IMAGES

Prescribed Placement for Premolar Bite-Wing Image

Center the receptor on the mandibular second premolar. The front edge of the receptor should be aligned with the midline of the mandibular canine. Make certain that the patient occlusal plane is parallel to the floor.

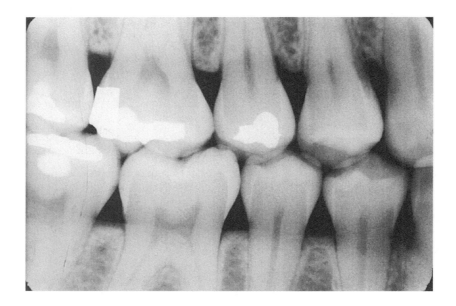

Prescribed Placement for Molar Bite-Wing Image

Center the receptor on the mandibular second molar. The front edge of the receptor should be aligned with the midline of the mandibular second premolar. Make certain that the patient occlusal plane is parallel to the floor.

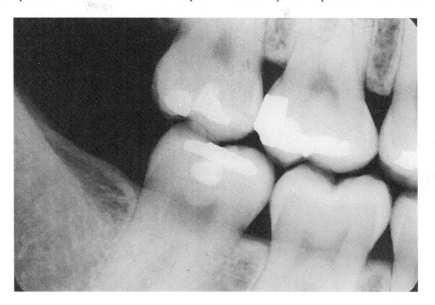

Exposure Sequence

Use the following exposure sequence for the bite-wing images:

1. right premolar

2. right molar

3. left premolar

4. left molar

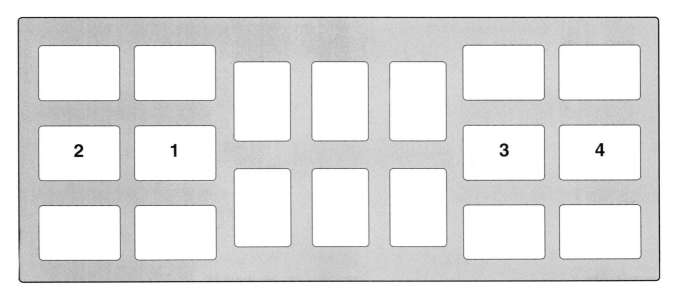

Module **6** Bite-Wing Technique with Tabs: Exposures, Mounting, and Critique

Equipment Needed

- radiology cubicle prepared with appropriate infection control protocol

- training manikin

- lead apron and thyroid collar

- size 2 receptors and tabs for bite-wing exposures in a plastic cup

- cotton rolls

Procedure

1. Set up DXTTR, utilizing the lead apron and thyroid collar.

2. Wash hands and don gloves.

3. Place receptors, cup, and cotton rolls on the covered work surface in a radiation-safe area, just outside the radiology cubicle.

4. Turn on the x-ray machine and set the exposure control panel to the appropriate setting for the premolar bite-wing projection.

5. Enter the radiology cubicle and move the tubehead into the area near the mandibular right premolar. Place the position indicating device (PID) as close to this anatomic area as possible *before* the receptor is inside the mouth.

6. Close the jaws of the training manikin together in a biting position. Set the vertical angulation of the PID at +10 degrees.

7. Stand in front of the manikin and place your index finger along the buccal surfaces of the premolar teeth. Align the end of the PID parallel to your finger and also parallel to the curvature of the arch. Direct the central ray through the contact areas of the premolar teeth (Fig. 6-2).

8. Over the covered work surface, place the tab against the receptor so that the receptor will be positioned horizontally in the mouth. The tab should be centered on the receptor.

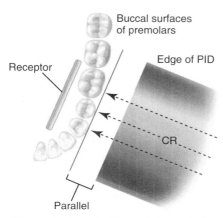

Fig. 6-2. The central ray is directed through the premolars.

9. Place the receptor with tab into the mouth of the teaching manikin, centered on tooth #29. Close training manikin carefully on the tab, ensuring that the distal aspect of tooth #27 is covered by the receptor. Align the PID to completely cover the receptor.

10. Expose the premolar bite-wing image.

11. Place the exposed receptor into a clean disposable cup in a radiation-safe area.

12. Move the tubehead into the area near the mandibular right molar. Place the PID as close to this anatomic area as possible *before* the receptor is inside the mouth.

13. Close the jaws of the training manikin together in a biting position. Set the vertical angulation of the PID at +10 degrees.

14. Stand in front of the manikin and place your index finger along the buccal surfaces of the molar teeth. Align the end of the PID parallel to your finger and also parallel to the curvature of the arch. Direct the central ray through the contact areas of the molar teeth (Fig. 6-3).

15. Over the covered work surface, place the tab against the receptor so that the receptor is positioned horizontally in the mouth. The tab should be centered on the receptor.

16. Place the receptor with tab into the mouth of the teaching manikin, centered on tooth #31. Close training manikin carefully on the tab, ensuring that the distal aspect of tooth #29 is covered by the receptor. Align the PID to completely cover the receptor.

17. Expose the molar bite-wing image.

18. Place the exposed receptor into a clean disposable cup in a radiation-safe area.

19. Continue with the bite-wing exposures according to the exposure sequence listed previously. Remember to adjust the control panel if necessary for premolar or molar exposures.

21. When all exposures are complete, remove gloves, wash your hands, and remove the lead apron and thyroid collar. Proceed to the darkroom or image retrieval area to process the radiographs.

22. Once all images have been retrieved, place in anatomic order with either a film mount or computer software. Evaluate your bite-wing exposures with the use of the image critique form on the next page. Note that only the bite-wing exposures should be evaluated at this time. When images are mounted and critiqued, inform the faculty to receive feedback.

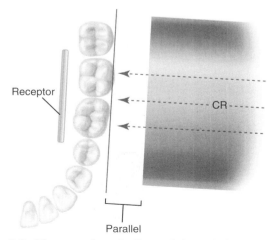

Fig. 6-3. The central ray is directed through the molar teeth.

Module 6   **Bite-Wing Technique with Tabs: Exposures, Mounting, and Critique**

Image Critique Form

Students: Evaluate the images created for this lab session. Use the letters in the Critique Key to describe errors seen on the images. Label each exposure with any errors seen.

Student Name: _____   Patient Name: _____   Date of Exam: _____   Grade: _____

Area Exposed	Student Evaluation of Error	Retakes* (Y)	Pt Management Issues* (need faculty signature)	Faculty Evaluation of Error*
Max Right Molar				
Max Right Premolar				
Max Right Canine				
Max Centrals				
Max Left Canine				
Max Left Premolar				
Max Left Molar				
Right Molar Bite-wing				
Right Premolar Bite-wing				
Left Premolar Bite-wing				
Left Molar Bite-wing				
Mand Right Molar				
Mand Right Premolar				
Mand Right Canine				
Mand Centrals				
Mand Left Canine				
Mand Left Premolar				
Mand Left Molar				
PANORAMIC RADIOGRAPH				

Critique Key

B = exposed backwards
C = cone-cut
E = elongation
F = foreshortening
FM = mounting error
H = horizontal angulation
IC = infection control error
LA = failure to place lead apron
M = movement
Ms = misc (specify)
P = receptor placement
PR = processing (specify)
R = retake (specify)
FP = Frankfort plane (up/down)
FT = focal trough (ant/post)
G = ghost image
MID = midsagittal plane
LAA = lead apron artifact

*Faculty: Review the images and critique as necessary; decide if retakes are necessary. Patient management issues may be documented in future semesters.

Module 6 **Bite-Wing Technique with Tabs: Exposures, Mounting, and Critique**

Image Critique Form

Students: Evaluate the images created for this lab session. Use the letters in the Critique Key to describe errors seen on the images. Label each exposure with any errors seen.

Student Name: _____ Patient Name: _____ Date of Exam: _____ Grade: _____

Area Exposed	Student Evaluation of Error	Retakes* (Y)	Pt Management Issues* (need faculty signature)	Faculty Evaluation of Error*	Critique Key
Max Right Molar					B = exposed backwards
Max Right Premolar					C = cone-cut
Max Right Canine					E = elongation
Max Centrals					F = foreshortening
Max Left Canine					FM = mounting error
Max Left Premolar					H = horizontal angulation
Max Left Molar					IC = infection control error
Right Molar Bite-wing					LA = failure to place lead apron
Right Premolar Bite-wing					M = movement
Left Premolar Bite-wing					Ms = misc (specify)
Left Molar Bite-wing					P = receptor placement
Mand Right Molar					PR = processing (specify)
Mand Right Premolar					R = retake (specify)
Mand Right Canine					FP = Frankfort plane (up/down)
Mand Centrals					FT = focal trough (ant/post)
Mand Left Canine					G = ghost image
Mand Left Premolar					MID = midsagittal plane
Mand Left Molar					LAA = lead apron artifact
PANORAMIC RADIOGRAPH					

*Faculty: Review the images and critique as necessary; decide if retakes are necessary. Patient management issues may be documented in future semesters.

Image Critique Form

Students: Evaluate the images created for this lab session. Use the letters in the Critique Key to describe errors seen on the images. Label each exposure with any errors seen.

Student Name: _____ Patient Name: _____ Date of Exam: _____ Grade: _____

Area Exposed	Student Evaluation of Error	Retakes* (Y)	Pt Management Issues* (need faculty signature)	Faculty Evaluation of Error*
Max Right Molar				
Max Right Premolar				
Max Right Canine				
Max Centrals				
Max Left Canine				
Max Left Premolar				
Max Left Molar				
Right Molar Bite-wing				
Right Premolar Bite-wing				
Left Premolar Bite-wing				
Left Molar Bite-wing				
Mand Right Molar				
Mand Right Premolar				
Mand Right Canine				
Mand Centrals				
Mand Left Canine				
Mand Left Premolar				
Mand Left Molar				
PANORAMIC RADIOGRAPH				

Critique Key

B = exposed backwards
C = cone-cut
E = elongation
F = foreshortening
FM = mounting error
H = horizontal angulation
IC = infection control error
LA = failure to place lead apron
M = movement
Ms = misc (specify)
P = receptor placement
PR = processing (specify)
R = retake (specify)
FP = Frankfort plane (up/down)
FT = focal trough (ant/post)
G = ghost image
MID = midsagittal plane
LAA = lead apron artifact

*Faculty: Review the images and critique as necessary; decide if retakes are necessary. Patient management issues may be documented in future semesters.

Module 6 Bite-Wing Technique with Tabs: Exposures, Mounting, and Critique

Image Critique Form

Students: Evaluate the images created for this lab session. Use the letters in the Critique Key to describe errors seen on the images. Label each exposure with any errors seen.

Student Name: _____   Patient Name: _____   Date of Exam: _____   Grade: _____

Area Exposed	Student Evaluation of Error	Retakes* (Y)	Pt Management Issues* (need faculty signature)	Faculty Evaluation of Error*
Max Right Molar				
Max Right Premolar				
Max Right Canine				
Max Centrals				
Max Left Canine				
Max Left Premolar				
Max Left Molar				
Right Molar Bite-wing				
Right Premolar Bite-wing				
Left Premolar Bite-wing				
Left Molar Bite-wing				
Mand Right Molar				
Mand Right Premolar				
Mand Right Canine				
Mand Centrals				
Mand Left Canine				
Mand Left Premolar				
Mand Left Molar				
PANORAMIC RADIOGRAPH				

Critique Key

B = exposed backwards
C = cone-cut
E = elongation
F = foreshortening
FM = mounting error
H = horizontal angulation
IC = infection control error
LA = failure to place lead apron
M = movement
Ms = misc (specify)
P = receptor placement
PR = processing (specify)
R = retake (specify)
FP = Frankfort plane (up/down)
FT = focal trough (ant/post)
G = ghost image
MID = midsagittal plane
LAA = lead apron artifact

*Faculty: Review the images and critique as necessary; decide if retakes are necessary. Patient management issues may be documented in future semesters.

CLINICAL LABORATORY ACTIVITY 6-1 WORKSHEET

Questions for Group Discussion

1. Which receptor placement is more difficult: maintaining the premolar receptor far enough forward to cover half of the mandibular canine *or* sustaining the molar placement far enough posteriorly to cover half of the mandibular second premolar?

   _____

   _____

   _____

2. Patients may grumble about the stiff edge of the receptor cutting into the soft tissue of the floor of the mouth. How do you accommodate this complaint?

   _____

   _____

   _____

3. Why is the bite-wing examination so common in dental offices?

   _____

   _____

   _____

4. What modifications are made if a child requires a bite-wing examination?

   _____

   _____

   _____

5. What modifications are made if your adult patient with a maxillary denture is prescribed bite-wing images?

   _____

   _____

   _____

Competency Examination: Bisecting Technique and Bite-Wing with Tabs Mounting and Critique

7

CRITERIA FOR COMPETENCY EXAMINATION

Student exposes 10 images on the RIGHT side of DXTTR in 30 minutes or less (the time limit is for exposures only, not processing or image retrieval). Student mounts the 10 images correctly.

The *10 exposures* include:

- four anterior periapical images exposed with the bisecting technique:

  - maxillary right canine
  - maxillary incisors

  - mandibular incisors
  - mandibular right canine

- four posterior periapical images exposed with the bisecting technique:

  - maxillary right premolar
  - maxillary right molar

  - mandibular right premolar
  - mandibular right molar

- two bite-wing (with tab) images:

  - right premolar and

  - right molar

After the images have been retrieved, the operator must correctly mount all 10 radiographs.
Grade is dependent on the following:

- lead apron/thyroid collar placement
- correct exposure sequence
- proper infection control procedures utilized
- correct exposure control settings chosen

- appropriate handling and use of teaching manikin
- diagnostic quality of the 10 images
- correct image mounting

A competency score of at least 75% is required to pass this examination. If the student does not reach a level of competency, it is at the discretion of the faculty whether the examination may be given a second time.

415

Image Critique Form: Bisecting, Bite-Wing with Tabs, Mounting

Students: Evaluate the images created for this lab session. Use the letters in the Critique Key to describe errors seen on the images. Label each exposure with any errors seen.

Student Name: _____   Patient Name: _____   Date of Exam: _____

Area Exposed	Student Evaluation of Error	Retakes (Y)	Pt Management Issues* (need faculty signature)	Faculty Evaluation of Error*
Max Right Molar				
Max Right Premolar				
Max Right Canine				
Max Centrals				
Max Left Canine				
Max Left Premolar				
Max Left Molar				
Right Molar Bite-wing				
Right Premolar Bite-wing				
Left Premolar Bite-wing				
Left Molar Bite-wing				
Mand Right Molar				
Mand Right Premolar				
Mand Right Canine				
Mand Centrals				
Mand Left Canine				
Mand Left Premolar				
Mand Left Molar				
PANORAMIC RADIOGRAPH				

Critique Key

B = exposed backwards
C = cone-cut
E = elongation
F = foreshortening
FM = mounting error
H = horizontal angulation
IC = infection control error
LA = failure to place lead apron
M = movement
Ms = misc (specify)
P = receptor placement
PR = processing (specify)
R = retake (specify)
FP = Frankfort plane (up/down)
FT = focal trough (ant/post)
G = ghost image
MID = midsagittal plane
LAA = lead apron artifact

Grade Achieved: _____   Faculty Signature: _____

*Faculty: Review the images and critique as necessary; decide if retakes are necessary. Patient management issues may be documented in future semesters.

Module **7** **Competency Examination: Bisecting Technique and Bite-Wing with Tabs Mounting and Critique**

Image Critique Form: Bisecting, Bite-Wing with Tabs, Mounting

Students: Evaluate the images created for this lab session. Use the letters in the Critique Key to describe errors seen on the images. Label each exposure with any errors seen.

Student Name: _____   Patient Name: _____   Date of Exam: _____

Area Exposed	Student Evaluation of Error	Retakes (Y)	Pt Management Issues* (need faculty signature)	Faculty Evaluation of Error*	Critique Key
Max Right Molar					B = exposed backwards
Max Right Premolar					C = cone-cut
Max Right Canine					E = elongation
Max Centrals					F = foreshortening
Max Left Canine					FM = mounting error
Max Left Premolar					H = horizontal angulation
Max Left Molar					IC = infection control error
Right Molar Bite-wing					LA = failure to place lead apron
Right Premolar Bite-wing					M = movement
Left Premolar Bite-wing					Ms = misc (specify)
Left Molar Bite-wing					P = receptor placement
Mand Right Molar					PR = processing (specify)
Mand Right Premolar					R = retake (specify)
Mand Right Canine					FP = Frankfort plane (up/down)
Mand Centrals					FT = focal trough (ant/post)
Mand Left Canine					G = ghost image
Mand Left Premolar					MID = midsagittal plane
Mand Left Molar					LAA = lead apron artifact
PANORAMIC RADIOGRAPH					

Grade Achieved: _____   Faculty Signature: _____

*Faculty: Review the images and critique as necessary; decide if retakes are necessary. Patient management issues may be documented in future semesters.

8 | Paralleling Technique

BASIC CONCEPTS OF THE PARALLELING TECHNIQUE

- The intraoral receptor is placed parallel to the long axis of the teeth being radiographed.

- The central ray is directed perpendicular to the receptor and long axis of the tooth.

- To achieve this result, a beam alignment device must be used.

CLINICAL LABORATORY ACTIVITY 8-1

Paralleling Technique: Anterior Region: Exposures, Mounting, Critique

Objectives

- Discuss the key terms associated with the paralleling technique: parallel, perpendicular, and intersecting.

- Illustrate the locations of the receptor, tooth, beam alignment device, and central ray.

- Describe the receptor size(s) used with the paralleling technique.

- Describe why a beam alignment device is required with the paralleling technique; demonstrate the assembly of the parts of the anterior XCP instruments.

- Describe patient and equipment preparations necessary before using the paralleling technique.

- List the correct sequence of exposure of the anterior projections.

- List the advantages and disadvantages of the paralleling technique.

Introduction

The goal of this laboratory exercise is to use the training manikin to produce diagnostic images of the maxillary and mandibular anterior teeth utilizing the paralleling technique with the XCP beam alignment devices. Depending on school policy, between six and seven total projections are exposed to cover the following areas: maxillary right and left canine, maxillary incisors, mandibular right and left canine, and mandibular incisors.

EXAMPLES OF MOUNTED DIAGNOSTIC ANTERIOR PERIAPICAL IMAGE

Maxillary Canine

- The entire crown and root of the canine, including the apex and the surrounding structures, must be visible.

- The interproximal alveolar bone and mesial contact of the canine must also be visible.

- The lingual cusp of the first premolar usually obscures the distal contact of the canine.

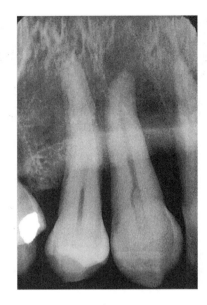

Maxillary Incisor

- The entire crowns and roots of one lateral and one central incisor, including the apices of the teeth and the surrounding structures, must be visible.

- The interproximal alveolar bone between the central and lateral and the mesial and distal contact areas, as well as the surrounding regions of bone, must also be visible.

- The mesial contact of the adjacent central incisor and the mesial contact of the adjacent canine should also be visible.

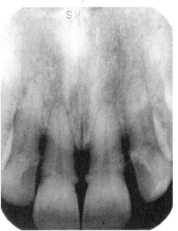

Mandibular Canine

- The entire crown and root of the canine, including the apex and the surrounding structures, must be visible.

- The interproximal alveolar bone and mesial and distal contacts must also be visible.

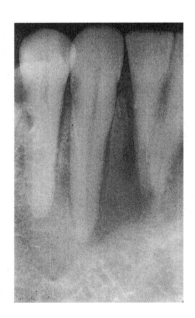

Mandibular Incisor

- The entire crowns and roots of the four mandibular incisors, including the apices of the teeth and the surrounding structures, must be visible.

- The contacts between the central incisors and those between the central and lateral incisors must also be visible.

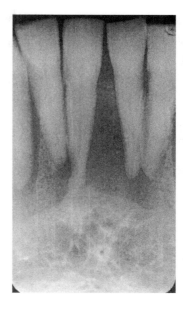

EXPOSURE SEQUENCE

Use the following exposure sequence for the anterior periapical images:

1. maxillary right canine

2. maxillary incisors

3. maxillary left canine

4. mandibular left canine

5. mandibular incisors

6. mandibular right canine

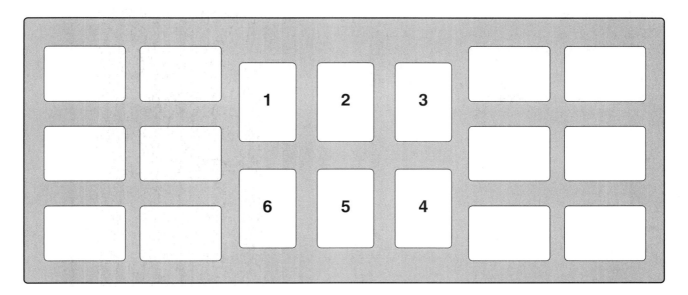

421

Equipment Needed

- radiology cubicle prepared with appropriate infection control protocol

- training manikin

- lead apron and thyroid collar

- size 1 and/or 2 receptors for anterior projections in a plastic cup

- beam alignment devices

- disposable bite blocks

- cotton rolls

Procedure

1. Set up DXTTR, utilizing the lead apron and thyroid collar.

2. Wash hands and don gloves.

3. Place receptors, cup, beam alignment devices, and cotton rolls on the covered work surface in a radiation-safe area, just outside the radiology cubicle.

4. Turn on the x-ray machine and set the exposure control panel to the appropriate setting for the maxillary canine projection.

5. Enter the radiology cubicle and move the tubehead into the area near the maxillary right canine. Place the position indicating device (PID) as close to this anatomic area as possible *before* the receptor is inside the mouth.

6. Over the covered work surface, assemble the anterior beam alignment device. Place the first receptor in a vertical direction snugly into the bite block.

7. Place the receptor and beam alignment device into the mouth of the teaching manikin, centered on tooth #6. Close training manikin carefully on the bite block. Align the PID with the anterior aiming ring of the beam alignment device.

8. Expose the periapical image.

9. Place the exposed receptor into a clean disposable cup in a radiation-safe area.

10. Continue to make exposures in the maxillary anterior region. Follow the exposure sequence listed previously. When the maxillary anterior teeth are complete, adjust the control panel if necessary for mandibular anterior exposures.

11. When all exposures are complete, remove gloves, wash your hands, and remove the lead apron and thyroid collar. Proceed to the darkroom or image retrieval area to process the radiographs.

12. Once all images have been retrieved, place in anatomic order with either a film mount or computer software. Evaluate your anterior exposures with the use of the image critique form on the next page. Note that only the anterior exposures should be evaluated at this time. When images are mounted and critiqued, inform the faculty to receive feedback.

Image Critique Form

Students: Evaluate the images created for this lab session. Use the letters in the Critique Key to describe errors seen on the images. Label each exposure with any errors seen.

Student Name: _____ Patient Name: _____ Date of Exam: _____ Grade: _____

Area Exposed	Student Evaluation of Error	Retakes* (Y)	Pt Management Issues* (need faculty signature)	Faculty Evaluation of Error*
Max Right Molar				
Max Right Premolar				
Max Right Canine				
Max Centrals				
Max Left Canine				
Max Left Premolar				
Max Left Molar				
Right Molar Bite-wing				
Right Premolar Bite-wing				
Left Premolar Bite-wing				
Left Molar Bite-wing				
Mand Right Molar				
Mand Right Premolar				
Mand Right Canine				
Mand Centrals				
Mand Left Canine				
Mand Left Premolar				
Mand Left Molar				
PANORAMIC RADIOGRAPH				

Critique Key

B = exposed backwards
C = cone-cut
E = elongation
F = foreshortening
FM = mounting error
H = horizontal angulation
IC = infection control error
LA = failure to place lead apron
M = movement
Ms = misc (specify)
P = receptor placement
PR = processing (specify)
R = retake (specify)
FP = Frankfort plane (up/down)
FT = focal trough (ant/post)
G = ghost image
MID = midsagittal plane
LAA = lead apron artifact

*Faculty: Review the images and critique as necessary; decide if retakes are necessary. Patient management issues may be documented in future semesters.

Image Critique Form

Students: Evaluate the images created for this lab session. Use the letters in the Critique Key to describe errors seen on the images. Label each exposure with any errors seen.

Student Name: _____   Patient Name: _____   Date of Exam: _____   Grade: _____

Area Exposed	Student Evaluation of Error	Retakes* (Y)	Pt Management Issues* (need faculty signature)	Faculty Evaluation of Error*
Max Right Molar				
Max Right Premolar				
Max Right Canine				
Max Centrals				
Max Left Canine				
Max Left Premolar				
Max Left Molar				
Right Molar Bite-wing				
Right Premolar Bite-wing				
Left Premolar Bite-wing				
Left Molar Bite-wing				
Mand Right Molar				
Mand Right Premolar				
Mand Right Canine				
Mand Centrals				
Mand Left Canine				
Mand Left Premolar				
Mand Left Molar				
PANORAMIC RADIOGRAPH				

Critique Key

B = exposed backwards
C = cone-cut
E = elongation
F = foreshortening
FM = mounting error
H = horizontal angulation
IC = infection control error
LA = failure to place lead apron
M = movement
Ms = misc (specify)
P = receptor placement
PR = processing (specify)
R = retake (specify)
FP = Frankfort plane (up/down)
FT = focal trough (ant/post)
G = ghost image
MID = midsagittal plane
LAA = lead apron artifact

*Faculty: Review the images and critique as necessary; decide if retakes are necessary. Patient management issues may be documented in future semesters.

Image Critique Form

Students: Evaluate the images created for this lab session. Use the letters in the Critique Key to describe errors seen on the images. Label each exposure with any errors seen.

Student Name: _____ Patient Name: _____ Date of Exam: _____ Grade: _____

Area Exposed	Student Evaluation of Error	Retakes* (Y)	Pt Management Issues* (need faculty signature)	Faculty Evaluation of Error*
Max Right Molar				
Max Right Premolar				
Max Right Canine				
Max Centrals				
Max Left Canine				
Max Left Premolar				
Max Left Molar				
Right Molar Bite-wing				
Right Premolar Bite-wing				
Left Premolar Bite-wing				
Left Molar Bite-wing				
Mand Right Molar				
Mand Right Premolar				
Mand Right Canine				
Mand Centrals				
Mand Left Canine				
Mand Left Premolar				
Mand Left Molar				
PANORAMIC RADIOGRAPH				

Critique Key

B = exposed backwards
C = cone-cut
E = elongation
F = foreshortening
FM = mounting error
H = horizontal angulation
IC = infection control error
LA = failure to place lead apron
M = movement
Ms = misc (specify)
P = receptor placement
PR = processing (specify)
R = retake (specify)
FP = Frankfort plane (up/down)
FT = focal trough (ant/post)
G = ghost image
MID = midsagittal plane
LAA = lead apron artifact

*Faculty: Review the images and critique as necessary; decide if retakes are necessary. Patient management issues may be documented in future semesters.

Image Critique Form

Students: Evaluate the images created for this lab session. Use the letters in the Critique Key to describe errors seen on the images. Label each exposure with any errors seen.

Student Name: _____ Patient Name: _____ Date of Exam: _____ Grade: _____

Area Exposed	Student Evaluation of Error	Retakes* (Y)	Pt Management Issues* (need faculty signature)	Faculty Evaluation of Error*
Max Right Molar				
Max Right Premolar				
Max Right Canine				
Max Centrals				
Max Left Canine				
Max Left Premolar				
Max Left Molar				
Right Molar Bite-wing				
Right Premolar Bite-wing				
Left Premolar Bite-wing				
Left Molar Bite-wing				
Mand Right Molar				
Mand Right Premolar				
Mand Right Canine				
Mand Centrals				
Mand Left Canine				
Mand Left Premolar				
Mand Left Molar				
PANORAMIC RADIOGRAPH				

Critique Key

B = exposed backwards
C = cone-cut
E = elongation
F = foreshortening
FM = mounting error
H = horizontal angulation
IC = infection control error
LA = failure to place lead apron
M = movement
Ms = misc (specify)
P = receptor placement
PR = processing (specify)
R = retake (specify)
FP = Frankfort plane (up/down)
FT = focal trough (ant/post)
G = ghost image
MID = midsagittal plane
LAA = lead apron artifact

*Faculty: Review the images and critique as necessary; decide if retakes are necessary. Patient management issues may be documented in future semesters.

CLINICAL LABORATORY ACTIVITY 8-1 WORKSHEET

Questions for Group Discussion

1. In what situations would the paralleling technique be preferred over the bisecting technique?

   _____

   _____

   _____

2. What was easy about using this intraoral radiographic technique? Why?

   _____

   _____

   _____

3. What was difficult about using this intraoral radiographic technique? Why?

   _____

   _____

   _____

4. Which anterior receptors are placed closer to the teeth, and which are placed farther away?

   _____

   _____

   _____

CLINICAL LABORATORY ACTIVITY 8-2

Paralleling Technique: Posterior Region: Exposures, Mounting, and Critique

Objectives

- Discuss the key terms associated with the paralleling technique: parallel, perpendicular, intersecting.

- Illustrate the location of the receptor, tooth, beam alignment device, and central ray.

- Describe the receptor size(s) used with the paralleling technique.

- Describe why a beam alignment device is required with the paralleling technique; demonstrate the assembly of the parts of the posterior XCP instruments.

- Explain why the posterior XCP instrument must be reassembled twice during exposures.

- Describe patient and equipment preparations necessary before using the paralleling technique.

- List the correct sequence of exposure of the posterior projections.

Introduction

The goal of this laboratory exercise is to produce diagnostic images with the training manikin of the maxillary and mandibular posterior teeth utilizing the paralleling technique with the XCP beam alignment devices. Eight total projections are exposed to cover the following areas: maxillary right and left premolar and molar regions, and mandibular right and left premolar and molar regions.

EXAMPLES OF MOUNTED DIAGNOSTIC POSTERIOR PERIAPICAL IMAGE

Maxillary Premolar

- All crowns and roots of the first and second premolars and of the first molar, including the apices, alveolar crests, contact areas, and surrounding bone, must be visible.

- The distal contact of the maxillary canine must also be visible.

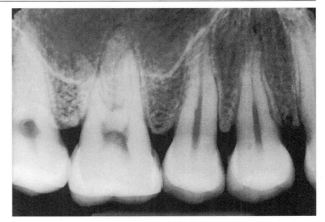

Maxillary Molar

- All crowns and roots of the first, second, and third molars, including the apices, alveolar crests, contact areas, surrounding bone, and tuberosity region, must be visible.

- The distal contact of the maxillary second premolar must also be visible.

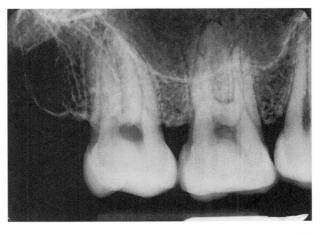

Mandibular Premolar

- All crowns and roots of the first and second premolars and of the first molar, including the apices, alveolar crests, contact areas, and surrounding bone, must be visible.

- The distal contact of the mandibular canine must also be visible.

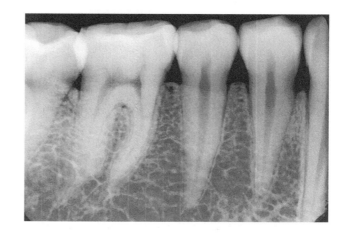

Mandibular Molar

- All crowns and roots of the first, second, and third molars, including the apices, alveolar crests, contact areas, and surrounding bone, must be visible.

- The distal contact of the mandibular second premolar must also be visible.

Exposure Sequence

Use the following exposure sequence for the posterior periapical images:

1. maxillary right premolar

2. maxillary right molar

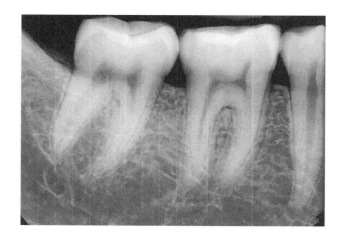

3. mandibular left premolar

4. mandibular left molar *(reassemble beam alignment device)*

5. maxillary left premolar

6. maxillary left molar

7. mandibular right premolar

8. mandibular right molar

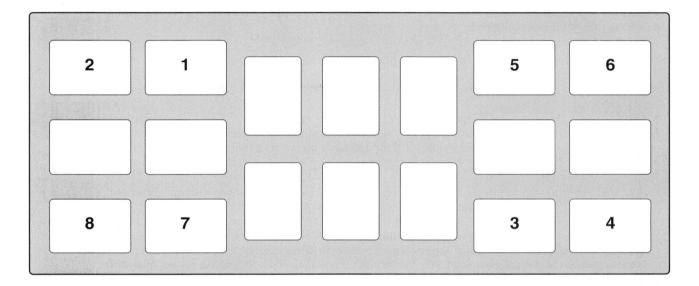

Equipment Needed

- radiology cubicle prepared with appropriate infection control protocol

- training manikin

- lead apron and thyroid collar

- receptors for posterior projections in a plastic cup

- beam alignment devices

- disposable bite blocks

- cotton rolls

Procedure

1. Set up DXTTR, utilizing the lead apron and thyroid collar.

2. Wash hands and don gloves.

3. Place receptors, cup, beam alignment devices, and cotton rolls on the covered work surface in a radiation-safe area, just outside the radiology cubicle.

4. Turn on the x-ray machine and set the exposure control panel to the appropriate setting for the maxillary premolar projection.

5. Enter the radiology cubicle and move the tubehead into the area near the maxillary right premolar. Place the PID as close to this anatomic area as possible *before* the receptor is inside the mouth.

6. Over the covered work surface, assemble the posterior beam alignment device. Place the first receptor in a horizontal direction snugly into the bite block.

7. Place the receptor and beam alignment device into the mouth of the teaching manikin, centered on teeth #4 and #5. Close training manikin carefully on the bite block. Align the PID with the posterior aiming ring of the beam alignment device.

8. Expose the periapical image.

9. Place the exposed receptor into a clean disposable cup in a radiation-safe area.

10. Continue to make exposures in the maxillary right posterior region. *Note:* To limit the number of times to readjust the beam alignment devices, follow the exposure sequence listed previously. Remember to adjust the control panel if necessary for maxillary premolar or molar exposures as well as for mandibular premolar or molar exposures.

11. When all exposures are complete, remove gloves, wash your hands, and remove the lead apron and thyroid collar. Proceed to the darkroom or image retrieval area to process the radiographs.

12. Once all images have been retrieved, place in anatomic order with either a film mount or computer software. Evaluate your posterior exposures with the use of the image critique form on the next page. Note that only the posterior exposures should be evaluated at this time. When images are mounted and critiqued, inform the faculty to receive feedback.

Image Critique Form

Students: Evaluate the images created for this lab session. Use the letters in the Critique Key to describe errors seen on the images. Label each exposure with any errors seen.

Student Name: _____   Patient Name: _____   Date of Exam: _____   Grade: _____

Area Exposed	Student Evaluation of Error	Retakes* (Y)	Pt Management Issues* (need faculty signature)	Faculty Evaluation of Error*
Max Right Molar				
Max Right Premolar				
Max Right Canine				
Max Centrals				
Max Left Canine				
Max Left Premolar				
Max Left Molar				
Right Molar Bite-wing				
Right Premolar Bite-wing				
Left Premolar Bite-wing				
Left Molar Bite-wing				
Mand Right Molar				
Mand Right Premolar				
Mand Right Canine				
Mand Centrals				
Mand Left Canine				
Mand Left Premolar				
Mand Left Molar				
PANORAMIC RADIOGRAPH				

Critique Key

B = exposed backwards
C = cone-cut
E = elongation
F = foreshortening
FM = mounting error
H = horizontal angulation
IC = infection control error
LA = failure to place lead apron
M = movement
Ms = misc (specify)
P = receptor placement
PR = processing (specify)
R = retake (specify)
FP = Frankfort plane (up/down)
FT = focal trough (ant/post)
G = ghost image
MID = midsagittal plane
LAA = lead apron artifact

*Faculty: Review the images and critique as necessary; decide if retakes are necessary. Patient management issues may be documented in future semesters.

Image Critique Form

Students: Evaluate the images created for this lab session. Use the letters in the Critique Key to describe errors seen on the images. Label each exposure with any errors seen.

Student Name: _____   Patient Name: _____   Date of Exam: _____   Grade: _____

Area Exposed	Student Evaluation of Error	Retakes* (Y)	Pt Management Issues* (need faculty signature)	Faculty Evaluation of Error*
Max Right Molar				
Max Right Premolar				
Max Right Canine				
Max Centrals				
Max Left Canine				
Max Left Premolar				
Max Left Molar				
Right Molar Bite-wing				
Right Premolar Bite-wing				
Left Premolar Bite-wing				
Left Molar Bite-wing				
Mand Right Molar				
Mand Right Premolar				
Mand Right Canine				
Mand Centrals				
Mand Left Canine				
Mand Left Premolar				
Mand Left Molar				
PANORAMIC RADIOGRAPH				

Critique Key

B = exposed backwards
C = cone-cut
E = elongation
F = foreshortening
FM = mounting error
H = horizontal angulation
IC = infection control error
LA = failure to place lead apron
M = movement
Ms = misc (specify)
P = receptor placement
PR = processing (specify)
R = retake (specify)
FP = Frankfort plane (up/down)
FT = focal trough (ant/post)
G = ghost image
MID = midsagittal plane
LAA = lead apron artifact

*Faculty: Review the images and critique as necessary; decide if retakes are necessary. Patient management issues may be documented in future semesters.

Image Critique Form

Students: Evaluate the images created for this lab session. Use the letters in the Critique Key to describe errors seen on the images. Label each exposure with any errors seen.

Student Name: _____ Patient Name: _____ Date of Exam: _____ Grade: _____

Area Exposed	Student Evaluation of Error	Retakes* (Y)	Pt Management Issues* (need faculty signature)	Faculty Evaluation of Error*
Max Right Molar				
Max Right Premolar				
Max Right Canine				
Max Centrals				
Max Left Canine				
Max Left Premolar				
Max Left Molar				
Right Molar Bite-wing				
Right Premolar Bite-wing				
Left Premolar Bite-wing				
Left Molar Bite-wing				
Mand Right Molar				
Mand Right Premolar				
Mand Right Canine				
Mand Centrals				
Mand Left Canine				
Mand Left Premolar				
Mand Left Molar				
PANORAMIC RADIOGRAPH				

Critique Key

B = exposed backwards
C = cone-cut
E = elongation
F = foreshortening
FM = mounting error
H = horizontal angulation
IC = infection control error
LA = failure to place lead apron
M = movement
Ms = misc (specify)
P = receptor placement
PR = processing (specify)
R = retake (specify)
FP = Frankfort plane (up/down)
FT = focal trough (ant/post)
G = ghost image
MID = midsagittal plane
LAA = lead apron artifact

*Faculty: Review the images and critique as necessary; decide if retakes are necessary. Patient management issues may be documented in future semesters.

Module **8** **Paralleling Technique**

Image Critique Form

Students: Evaluate the images created for this lab session. Use the letters in the Critique Key to describe errors seen on the images. Label each exposure with any errors seen.

Student Name: _____ Patient Name: _____ Date of Exam: _____ Grade: _____

Area Exposed	Student Evaluation of Error	Retakes* (Y)	Pt Management Issues* (need faculty signature)	Faculty Evaluation of Error*	Critique Key
Max Right Molar					B = exposed backwards
Max Right Premolar					C = cone-cut
Max Right Canine					E = elongation
Max Centrals					F = foreshortening
Max Left Canine					FM = mounting error
Max Left Premolar					H = horizontal angulation
Max Left Molar					IC = infection control error
Right Molar Bite-wing					LA = failure to place lead apron
Right Premolar Bite-wing					M = movement
Left Premolar Bite-wing					Ms = misc (specify)
Left Molar Bite-wing					P = receptor placement
Mand Right Molar					PR = processing (specify)
Mand Right Premolar					R = retake (specify)
Mand Right Canine					FP = Frankfort plane (up/down)
Mand Centrals					FT = focal trough (ant/post)
Mand Left Canine					G = ghost image
Mand Left Premolar					MID = midsagittal plane
Mand Left Molar					LAA = lead apron artifact
PANORAMIC RADIOGRAPH					

*Faculty: Review the images and critique as necessary; decide if retakes are necessary. Patient management issues may be documented in future semesters.

CLINICAL LABORATORY ACTIVITY 8-2 WORKSHEET

Questions for Group Discussion

1. Why is it recommended that the bite block be placed against the occlusal surfaces of the teeth being radiographed *before* instructing the patient to bite?

   _____

   _____

   _____

2. Patients may close their lips together but not completely occlude on the bite block for comfort reasons. Why is this not recommended? How would the operator know if this is happening?

   _____

   _____

   _____

3. How would the operator accommodate the presence of maxillary torus or mandibular tori?

   _____

   _____

   _____

4. What instructions should be given about the patient's tongue during mandibular posterior exposures?

   _____

   _____

   _____

437

CLINICAL LABORATORY ACTIVITY 8-3

Paralleling Technique: Bite-Wing Images

Objectives

- Illustrate the locations of the receptor, tooth, beam alignment device, and central ray for both premolar and molar placements.

- Describe the receptor size used with the bite-wing technique.

- Demonstrate the assembly of the parts of the XCP instrument for the bite-wing exposure.

- Describe patient and equipment preparations necessary before using the bite-wing technique.

- List the correct sequence of exposure of the premolar and molar projections; state the correct sequence when the bite-wing exposures are part of a full-mouth series.

Introduction

The goal of this laboratory exercise is to use the training manikin to produce diagnostic images of the maxillary and mandibular posterior teeth utilizing the bite-wing technique with the XCP beam alignment devices (Fig. 8-1). Four total projections are exposed to cover the following areas: right and left premolar and molar regions.

BASIC CONCEPTS OF THE BITE-WING TECHNIQUE

- Place the receptor in the mouth parallel to the crowns of the maxillary and mandibular posterior teeth.

- Center the bite block on the occlusal surfaces of the mandibular premolar and molar teeth.

- The patient bites on the bite block of the bite-wing beam alignment device.

- The vertical and horizontal angulation is determined by the beam alignment device and proper PID position.

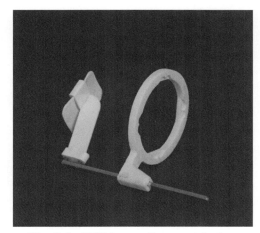

Fig. 8-1. XCP beam alignment device.

Prescribed Placement for Premolar Bite-Wing Image

Center the receptor on the mandibular second premolar. The front edge of the receptor should be aligned with the midline of the mandibular canine. Make certain that the patient occlusal plane is parallel to the floor.

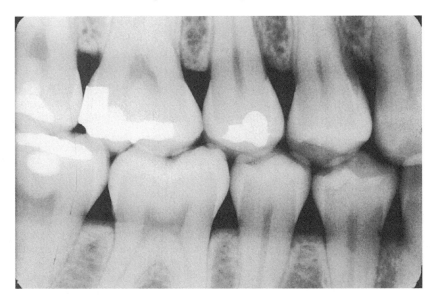

Prescribed Placement for Molar Bite-Wing Image

Center the receptor on the mandibular second molar. The front edge of the receptor should be aligned with the midline of the mandibular second premolar. Make certain that the patient occlusal plane is parallel to the floor.

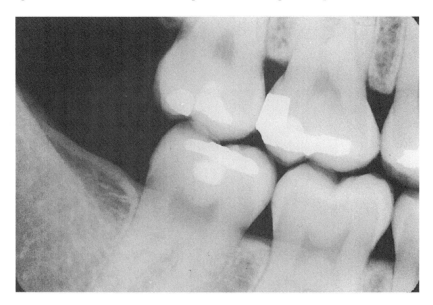

Exposure Sequence

Use the following exposure sequence for the bite-wing images:

1. right premolar

2. right molar

3. left premolar

4. left molar

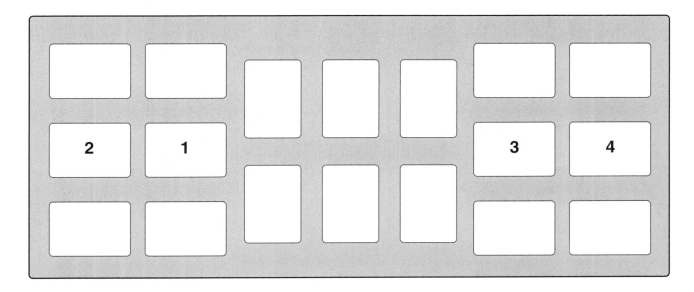

Equipment Needed

- radiology cubicle prepared with appropriate infection control protocol

- training manikin

- lead apron and thyroid collar

- Size 1 and/or 2 receptors in a plastic cup

- beam alignment devices

- disposable bite blocks

- cotton rolls

Procedure

1. Set up DXTTR, utilizing the lead apron and thyroid collar.

2. Wash hands and don gloves.

3. Place receptors and cup on the covered work surface in a radiation-safe area, just outside the radiology cubicle.

4. Turn on the x-ray machine and set the exposure control panel to the appropriate setting for the premolar bite-wing projection.

5. Enter the radiology cubicle and move the tubehead into the area near the mandibular right premolar. Place the PID as close to this anatomic area as possible *before* the receptor is inside the mouth.

6. Over the covered work surface, assemble the bite-wing beam alignment device. Place the first receptor in a horizontal direction snugly into the bite block.

7. Place the receptor and beam alignment device into the mouth of the teaching manikin, centered on tooth #29.

8. Close training manikin carefully on the bite block, ensuring that the distal aspect of tooth #27 is covered by the receptor. Align the PID with the bite-wing aiming ring of the beam alignment device.

9. Expose the premolar bite-wing image.

10. Place the exposed receptor into a clean disposable cup in a radiation-safe area.

11. Place the second receptor in a horizontal direction snugly into the bite block.

12. Place the receptor and beam alignment device into the mouth of the teaching manikin, centered on tooth #31.

13. Close training manikin carefully on the bite block, ensuring that the distal of tooth #29 is covered by the receptor. Align the PID with the bite-wing aiming ring of the beam alignment device.

14. Expose the molar bite-wing image.

15. Place the exposed receptor into a clean disposable cup in a radiation-safe area.

16. Continue with the bite-wing exposures according to the exposure sequence listed previously. Remember to adjust the control panel if necessary for premolar or molar exposures.

17. When all exposures are complete, remove gloves, wash your hands, and remove the lead apron and thyroid collar. Proceed to the darkroom or image retrieval area to process the radiographs.

18. Once all images have been retrieved, place in anatomic order with either a film mount or computer software. Evaluate your bite-wing exposures with the use of the image critique form on the next page. Note that only the bite-wing exposures should be evaluated at this time. When images are mounted and critiqued, inform the faculty to receive feedback.

Image Critique Form

Students: Evaluate the images created for this lab session. Use the letters in the Critique Key to describe errors seen on the images. Label each exposure with any errors seen.

Student Name: _____   Patient Name: _____   Date of Exam: _____   Grade: _____

Critique Key

B = exposed backwards
C = cone-cut
E = elongation
F = foreshortening
FM = mounting error
H = horizontal angulation
IC = infection control error
LA = failure to place lead apron
M = movement
Ms = misc (specify)
P = receptor placement
PR = processing (specify)
R = retake (specify)
FP = Frankfort plane (up/down)
FT = focal trough (ant/post)
G = ghost image
MID = midsagittal plane
LAA = lead apron artifact

Area Exposed	Student Evaluation of Error	Retakes* (Y)	Pt Management Issues* (need faculty signature)	Faculty Evaluation of Error*
Max Right Molar				
Max Right Premolar				
Max Right Canine				
Max Centrals				
Max Left Canine				
Max Left Premolar				
Max Left Molar				
Right Molar Bite-wing				
Right Premolar Bite-wing				
Left Premolar Bite-wing				
Left Molar Bite-wing				
Mand Right Molar				
Mand Right Premolar				
Mand Right Canine				
Mand Centrals				
Mand Left Canine				
Mand Left Premolar				
Mand Left Molar				
PANORAMIC RADIOGRAPH				

*Faculty: Review the images and critique as necessary; decide if retakes are necessary. Patient management issues may be documented in future semesters.

Image Critique Form

Students: Evaluate the images created for this lab session. Use the letters in the Critique Key to describe errors seen on the images. Label each exposure with any errors seen.

Student Name: _____ Patient Name: _____ Date of Exam: _____ Grade: _____

Area Exposed	Student Evaluation of Error	Retakes* (Y)	Pt Management Issues* (need faculty signature)	Faculty Evaluation of Error*
Max Right Molar				
Max Right Premolar				
Max Right Canine				
Max Centrals				
Max Left Canine				
Max Left Premolar				
Max Left Molar				
Right Molar Bite-wing				
Right Premolar Bite-wing				
Left Premolar Bite-wing				
Left Molar Bite-wing				
Mand Right Molar				
Mand Right Premolar				
Mand Right Canine				
Mand Centrals				
Mand Left Canine				
Mand Left Premolar				
Mand Left Molar				
PANORAMIC RADIOGRAPH				

Critique Key

B = exposed backwards
C = cone-cut
E = elongation
F = foreshortening
FM = mounting error
H = horizontal angulation
IC = infection control error
LA = failure to place lead apron
M = movement
Ms = misc (specify)
P = receptor placement
PR = processing (specify)
R = retake (specify)
FP = Frankfort plane (up/down)
FT = focal trough (ant/post)
G = ghost image
MID = midsagittal plane
LAA = lead apron artifact

*Faculty: Review the images and critique as necessary; decide if retakes are necessary. Patient management issues may be documented in future semesters.

Image Critique Form

Students: Evaluate the images created for this lab session. Use the letters in the Critique Key to describe errors seen on the images. Label each exposure with any errors seen.

Student Name: _____   Patient Name: _____   Date of Exam: _____   Grade: _____

Area Exposed	Student Evaluation of Error	Retakes* (Y)	Pt Management Issues* (need faculty signature)	Faculty Evaluation of Error*
Max Right Molar				
Max Right Premolar				
Max Right Canine				
Max Centrals				
Max Left Canine				
Max Left Premolar				
Max Left Molar				
Right Molar Bite-wing				
Right Premolar Bite-wing				
Left Premolar Bite-wing				
Left Molar Bite-wing				
Mand Right Molar				
Mand Right Premolar				
Mand Right Canine				
Mand Centrals				
Mand Left Canine				
Mand Left Premolar				
Mand Left Molar				
PANORAMIC RADIOGRAPH				

Critique Key

B = exposed backwards
C = cone-cut
E = elongation
F = foreshortening
FM = mounting error
H = horizontal angulation
IC = infection control error
LA = failure to place lead apron
M = movement
Ms = misc (specify)
P = receptor placement
PR = processing (specify)
R = retake (specify)
FP = Frankfort plane (up/down)
FT = focal trough (ant/post)
G = ghost image
MID = midsagittal plane
LAA = lead apron artifact

*Faculty: Review the images and critique as necessary; decide if retakes are necessary. Patient management issues may be documented in future semesters.

Image Critique Form

Students: Evaluate the images created for this lab session. Use the letters in the Critique Key to describe errors seen on the images. Label each exposure with any errors seen.

Student Name: _____   Patient Name: _____   Date of Exam: _____   Grade: _____

Area Exposed	Student Evaluation of Error	Retakes* (Y)	Pt Management Issues* (need faculty signature)	Faculty Evaluation of Error*
Max Right Molar				
Max Right Premolar				
Max Right Canine				
Max Centrals				
Max Left Canine				
Max Left Premolar				
Max Left Molar				
Right Molar Bite-wing				
Right Premolar Bite-wing				
Left Premolar Bite-wing				
Left Molar Bite-wing				
Mand Right Molar				
Mand Right Premolar				
Mand Right Canine				
Mand Centrals				
Mand Left Canine				
Mand Left Premolar				
Mand Left Molar				
PANORAMIC RADIOGRAPH				

Critique Key

B = exposed backwards
C = cone-cut
E = elongation
F = foreshortening
FM = mounting error
H = horizontal angulation
IC = infection control error
LA = failure to place lead apron
M = movement
Ms = misc (specify)
P = receptor placement
PR = processing (specify)
R = retake (specify)
FP = Frankfort plane (up/down)
FT = focal trough (ant/post)
G = ghost image
MID = midsagittal plane
LAA = lead apron artifact

*Faculty: Review the images and critique as necessary; decide if retakes are necessary. Patient management issues may be documented in future semesters.

CLINICAL LABORATORY ACTIVITY 8-3 WORKSHEET

1. Why is it recommended that the bite block be placed against the occlusal surfaces of the mandibular teeth (instead of the maxillary teeth) *before* instructing the patient to bite?

   _____

   _____

   _____

2. When mounting a full-mouth series, why is it suggested to mount the bite-wing images first?

   _____

   _____

   _____

3. Why does the error of horizontal overlap still occur on bite-wing images produced with the beam alignment device?

   _____

   _____

   _____

4. What modifications would be made if the patient is missing one of the teeth discussed in receptor placement, such as tooth #29?

   _____

   _____

   _____

Competency Examination: Paralleling Technique: Periapical and Bite-Wing Mounting and Critique

9

CRITERIA FOR COMPETENCY EXAMINATION

Student exposes *10* images on the LEFT side of DXTTR in 30 minutes or less (the time limit is for exposures only, not processing or image retrieval). Student mounts the 10 images correctly.

The *10 exposures* include:

- four anterior periapical images exposed with the paralleling technique:

  - maxillary left canine
  - maxillary incisors
  - mandibular incisors
  - mandibular left canine

- four posterior periapical images exposed with the paralleling technique:

  - maxillary left premolar
  - maxillary left molar
  - mandibular left premolar
  - mandibular left molar

- two bite-wing images exposed with the paralleling technique:

  - left premolar and
  - left molar

After the images have been retrieved, the operator must correctly mount all 10 radiographs. Grade is dependent on the following:

- lead apron/thyroid collar placement
- correct exposure sequence
- proper infection control procedures utilized
- correct exposure control settings chosen
- correct beam alignment device assembly
- appropriate handling and use of teaching manikin
- diagnostic quality of the 10 images
- correct image mounting

A competency score of at least 75% is required to pass this examination. If the student does not reach a level of competency, it is at the discretion of the faculty whether the examination may be given a second time.

Image Critique Form: Paralleling Critique

Students: Evaluate the images created for this lab session. Use the letters in the Critique Key to describe errors seen on the images. Label each exposure with any errors seen.

Student Name: _____

Patient Name: _____

Date of Exam: _____

Area Exposed	Student Evaluation of Error	Retakes (Y)	Pt Management Issues* (need faculty signature)	Faculty Evaluation of Error*	Critique Key
Max Right Molar					B = exposed backwards
Max Right Premolar					C = cone-cut
Max Right Canine					E = elongation
Max Centrals					F = foreshortening
Max Left Canine					FM = mounting error
Max Left Premolar					H = horizontal angulation
Max Left Molar					IC = infection control error
Right Molar Bite-wing					LA = failure to place lead apron
Right Premolar Bite-wing					M = movement
Left Premolar Bite-wing					Ms = misc (specify)
Left Molar Bite-wing					P = receptor placement
Mand Right Molar					PR = processing (specify)
Mand Right Premolar					R = retake (specify)
Mand Right Canine					FP = Frankfort plane (up/down)
Mand Centrals					FT = focal trough (ant/post)
Mand Left Canine					G = ghost image
Mand Left Premolar					MID = midsagittal plane
Mand Left Molar					LAA = lead apron artifact
PANORAMIC RADIOGRAPH					

Grade Achieved: _____

Faculty Signature: _____

*Faculty: Review the images and critique as necessary; decide if retakes are necessary. Patient management issues may be documented in future semesters.

451

Image Critique Form: Paralleling Critique

Students: Evaluate the images created for this lab session. Use the letters in the Critique Key to describe errors seen on the images. Label each exposure with any errors seen.

Student Name: _____   Patient Name: _____   Date of Exam: _____

Area Exposed	Student Evaluation of Error	Retakes (Y)	Pt Management Issues* (need faculty signature)	Faculty Evaluation of Error*
Max Right Molar				
Max Right Premolar				
Max Right Canine				
Max Centrals				
Max Left Canine				
Max Left Premolar				
Max Left Molar				
Right Molar Bite-wing				
Right Premolar Bite-wing				
Left Premolar Bite-wing				
Left Molar Bite-wing				
Mand Right Molar				
Mand Right Premolar				
Mand Right Canine				
Mand Centrals				
Mand Left Canine				
Mand Left Premolar				
Mand Left Molar				
PANORAMIC RADIOGRAPH				

Critique Key

B = exposed backwards
C = cone-cut
E = elongation
F = foreshortening
FM = mounting error
H = horizontal angulation
IC = infection control error
LA = failure to place lead apron
M = movement
Ms = misc (specify)
P = receptor placement
PR = processing (specify)
R = retake (specify)
FP = Frankfort plane (up/down)
FT = focal trough (ant/post)
G = ghost image
MID = midsagittal plane
LAA = lead apron artifact

Grade Achieved: _____   Faculty Signature: _____

*Faculty: Review the images and critique as necessary; decide if retakes are necessary. Patient management issues may be documented in future semesters.

452

10 | Occlusal Technique

BASIC CONCEPTS OF THE OCCLUSAL TECHNIQUE

- The occlusal technique is a supplementary intraoral technique used when larger areas of the maxilla and mandible must be visualized.
- Place the receptor in the mouth between the occlusal surfaces of the maxillary and mandibular teeth; ensure that the correct side of the receptor is facing the tubehead.
- The patient gently bites on the surface of the receptor.
- The vertical angulation will be determined by the region of interest being examined.

CLINICAL LABORATORY ACTIVITY 10-1
Occlusal Technique

Objectives

- Illustrate the location of the receptor, teeth, and central ray for the maxillary and mandibular occlusal placements.
- Describe the receptor size used with the occlusal technique for adults and children.
- Describe patient and equipment preparations necessary before using the occlusal technique, including the appropriate vertical angulations for the maxillary and mandibular occlusal images.

Introduction

The goal of this laboratory exercise is to use the training manikin to produce diagnostic images of the maxillary and mandibular arches utilizing the occlusal technique. Four total occlusal projections are exposed: two in the maxillary arch and two in the mandibular arch.

EXAMPLES OF MOUNTED DIAGNOSTIC OCCLUSAL IMAGES

Prescribed Placement for Maxillary Topographic Occlusal Image

Position the size 4 receptor in the mouth with the appropriate side of the receptor facing the maxillary arch. (Please note: Size 2 receptor may be used if working with a younger patient.) The longer edge of the receptor should be placed in a side-to-side direction intraorally. Insert the receptor as far posteriorly as the patient's anatomy permits. Instruct the patient to bite gently on the surface of the receptor to stabilize it for exposure.

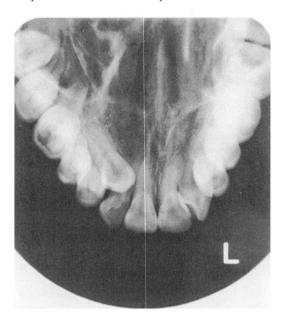

Prescribed Placement for Maxillary Lateral Occlusal Image

Position the size 4 receptor in the mouth with the appropriate side of the receptor facing the maxillary arch. The longer edge of the receptor should be placed in a side-to-side direction intraorally. Insert the receptor as far posteriorly as the patient's anatomy permits. Shift the receptor to the right or left side (depending on the region of interest) of the maxilla to extend approximately ½ inch beyond the buccal surfaces of the maxillary posterior teeth. Instruct the patient to bite gently on the surface of the receptor to stabilize it for exposure.

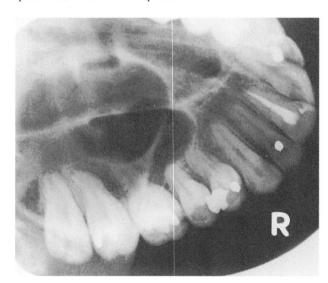

Prescribed Placement for Mandibular Topographic Occlusal Image

Position the size 4 receptor in the mouth with the appropriate side of the receptor facing the mandibular arch. The longer edge of the receptor should be placed in a side-to-side direction intraorally. Insert the receptor as far posteriorly as the patient's anatomy permits. Instruct the patient to bite gently on the surface of the receptor to stabilize it for exposure.

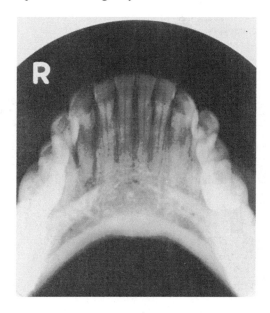

Prescribed Placement for Mandibular Cross-Sectional Occlusal Image

The patient is placed in a supine posture. Position the size 4 receptor in the mouth with the appropriate side of the receptor facing the mandibular arch. The longer edge of the receptor should be placed in a side-to-side direction intraorally. Insert the receptor as far posteriorly as the patient's anatomy permits. Instruct the patient to bite gently on the surface of the receptor to stabilize it for exposure.

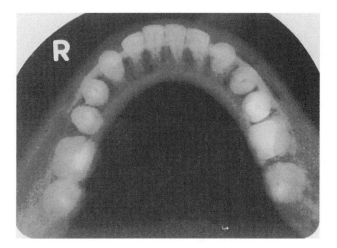

Exposure Sequence

Use the following exposure sequence for the occlusal images:

1. maxillary topographic

2. maxillary lateral

3. mandibular topographic

4. mandibular cross-sectional

Equipment Needed

- radiology cubicle prepared with appropriate infection control protocol

- training manikin

- lead apron and thyroid collar

- receptors in a plastic cup (size 4 receptors for adult patients; size 2 receptors for children)

Procedure

1. Set up DXTTR, utilizing the lead apron and thyroid collar.

2. Wash hands and don gloves.

3. Place receptors and cup on the covered work surface in a radiation-safe area, just outside the radiology cubicle.

4. Turn on the x-ray machine and set the exposure control panel to the appropriate setting for the maxillary occlusal projection.

5. Enter the radiology cubicle and move the tubehead into the area near the maxillary or mandibular arch. Place the position indicating device (PID) as close as possible to the assigned anatomic area *before* the receptor is inside the mouth.

6. Retrieve the receptor from the covered work surface.

Maxillary Topographic

7. Make certain the maxillary arch of the teaching manikin is parallel to the floor.

8. Place the receptor into the mouth of the teaching manikin with the longer edge of the receptor in a side-to-side direction. Gently guide the receptor as far posteriorly as possible keeping it centered in the mouth. Close manikin carefully on the receptor.

9. Position the PID with the central ray directed toward the center of the receptor using a vertical angulation of +65 degrees (the top edge of the PID is usually close in proximity to the bridge of the nose and the area between the eyebrows).

10. Expose the occlusal image.

11. Place the exposed receptor into a clean disposable cup in a radiation-safe area.

Maxillary Lateral

12. Make certain the maxillary arch of the teaching manikin is parallel to the floor.

13. Place the receptor into the mouth of the teaching manikin with the longer edge of the receptor in a side-to-side direction. Gently guide the receptor as far posteriorly as possible. Shift the receptor to the right side of the arch so that it extends approximately ½ inch beyond the buccal surfaces of the right posterior teeth. Close manikin carefully on the receptor.

14. Position the PID with the central ray directed toward the center of the receptor using a vertical angulation of +60 degrees (the top edge of the PID is usually close in proximity to the outer corner of the right eyebrow with the central ray directed toward the zygomatic arch).

15. Expose the occlusal image.

16. Place the exposed receptor into a clean disposable cup in a radiation-safe area.

Mandibular Topographic

17. Check the exposure control panel for the appropriate setting for the mandibular occlusal projections.

18. Make certain the mandibular arch of the teaching manikin is parallel to the floor. Reclining the manikin in a semi-supine position (or tipping the dental chair back) may be recommended if it is difficult to set the PID at -55 degrees. However, the vertical angulation will change if the occlusal plane of the patient is not parallel to the floor.

19. Place the receptor into the mouth of the teaching manikin with the longer edge of the receptor in a side-to-side direction. Gently guide the receptor as far posteriorly as possible keeping it centered in the mouth. Close manikin carefully on the receptor.

20. Position the PID with the central ray directed toward the center of the receptor using a vertical angulation of −55 degrees (the PID is usually centered over the area of the chin).

21. Expose the occlusal image.

22. Place the exposed receptor into a clean disposable cup in a radiation-safe area.

Mandibular Cross-Sectional

23. Make certain the mandibular arch of the teaching manikin is *perpendicular* to the floor. Reclining the manikin in a supine position is recommended. In addition, ensure that the thyroid collar is not blocking any portion of the x-ray beam.

24. Place the receptor into the mouth of the teaching manikin with the longer edge of the receptor in a side-to-side direction. Gently guide the receptor as far posteriorly as possible, keeping it centered in the mouth. Close manikin carefully on the receptor.

25. Position the PID with the central ray directed toward the center of the receptor using a vertical angulation of 90 degrees (the PID is usually centered approximately one inch below the area of the chin).

26. Expose the occlusal image.

27. Place the exposed receptor into a clean disposable cup in a radiation-safe area.

28. Once all images have been retrieved, place in exposure order with either a film mount or computer software. Evaluate your exposures with the use of the image critique form on the next page. Note that only occlusal images should be evaluated at this time. When images have been critiqued, inform the faculty to receive feedback.

Image Critique Form

Students: Evaluate the images created for this lab session. Use the letters in the Critique Key to describe errors seen on the images. Label each exposure with any errors seen.

Student Name: _____   Patient Name: _____   Date of Exam: _____   Grade: _____

Area Exposed	Student Evaluation of Error	Retakes* (Y)	Pt Management Issues* (need faculty signature)	Faculty Evaluation of Error*	Critique Key
Maxillary topographic					B = exposed backwards
Maxillary lateral occlusal					C = cone-cut
Mandibular topographic					E = elongation
Mandibular cross-sectional					F = foreshortening
					IC = infection control error
					LA = failure to place lead apron
					M = movement
					Ms = misc (specify)
					P = receptor placement
					PR = processing (specify)
					R = retake (specify)

*Faculty: Review the images and critique as necessary; decide if retakes are necessary. Patient management issues may be documented in future semesters.

Image Critique Form

Students: Evaluate the images created for this lab session. Use the letters in the Critique Key to describe errors seen on the images. Label each exposure with any errors seen.

Student Name: _____   Patient Name: _____   Date of Exam: _____   Grade: _____

Area Exposed	Student Evaluation of Error	Retakes* (Y)	Pt Management Issues* (need faculty signature)	Faculty Evaluation of Error*
Maxillary topographic				
Maxillary lateral occlusal				
Mandibular topographic				
Mandibular cross-sectional				

Critique Key

B = exposed backwards
C = cone-cut
E = elongation
F = foreshortening
IC = infection control error
LA = failure to place lead apron
M = movement
Ms = misc (specify)
P = receptor placement
PR = processing (specify)
R = retake (specify)

*Faculty: Review the images and critique as necessary; decide if retakes are necessary. Patient management issues may be documented in future semesters.

Name _____

Date _____

CLINICAL LABORATORY ACTIVITY 10-1 WORKSHEET

Questions for Group Discussion

1. List several clinical conditions where an occlusal image might be prescribed for an adult patient. List several for the child patient.

   _____

   _____

   _____

2. Your patient has a fractured mandible and can barely open his or her mouth. Explain how you would position him or her for the exposure of a mandibular cross-sectional occlusal image.

   _____

   _____

   _____

3. What does the term "topographic" refer to? Why is this term used to describe several of the occlusal images you exposed?

   _____

   _____

   _____

4. Your patient is an edentulous adult. Should you leave the dentures in place for the exposure of maxillary and mandibular occlusal images?

   _____

   _____

   _____

5. A cone-cut error is always seen when size 4 receptors are used in occlusal imaging. Should the cone-cut error be seen when a size 2 receptor is used?

   _____

   _____

   _____

461

Practice with Peer Patients

INTRODUCTION

The goal of this laboratory exercise is to reinforce material learned with the training manikin and apply the concepts to working with peer patients. The student will have the opportunity to practice the following intraoral techniques *without exposure:*

1. bisecting
2. bite-wing with tabs
3. paralleling
4. occlusal

REMINDERS

- **No exposures are to be made!**
- Infection control protocol must be strictly observed!
- Examine inside your patient's mouth before beginning any procedures. Perform a quick oral examination to see the oral cavity before receptor placement. Observe such findings as small mouths with limited opening, mandibular tori, maxillary torus, number of teeth present, missing teeth, and so on.
- Limit the amount of time the receptor is inside the mouth. To do this, make certain that the correct exposure setting is chosen before receptor placement. In addition, move the position indicating device (PID) to the prescribed anatomic area before receptor placement.
- Place the receptor carefully. Intraoral tissues are much more fragile than the teaching manikin. If the peer patient is struggling, remove the receptor and pause for a moment or two.
- Students should rotate and change partners as much as time allows to work with a variety of oral cavities.
- Have a positive and confident attitude!

Reminders for the Bisecting Technique

- Picture the placement of the receptor inside the mouth, and try to visualize the imaginary angle created between the receptor and the tooth. Align the PID to bisect the imaginary line created between the receptor and tooth. The central ray of radiation should be directed at a 90-degree angle to the imaginary bisector.
- Also, try to visualize the central ray directed through the teeth, opening up the contact areas. Place the PID as close to these correct settings as possible *before* the receptor is inside the mouth.
- Center the bite block on the teeth being radiographed.

Reminders for the Bite-Wing with Tab Technique

- Instruct your patient to close his or her teeth together in a biting position. Set the vertical angulation of the PID at +10 degrees.

- Stand in front of the patient and place your index finger along the buccal surfaces of the premolar teeth. Align the end of the PID parallel to your finger and also parallel to the curvature of the arch. Direct the central ray through the contact areas of the premolar teeth (Figure 11-1).

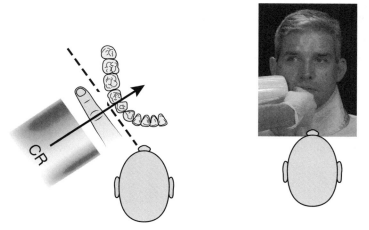

Fig. 11-1. Alignment of the bite-wing with tab technique.

- Align the molar bite-wing in the same way, lining up the PID before receptor placement in the mouth.

Reminders for the Paralleling Technique

- Assemble the beam alignment devices ahead of time, over the covered work surface. Place the receptors snugly into the bite block.

- Carefully place the receptor and beam alignment device into the patient's mouth, centered on the prescribed teeth. Place the bite block against the incisal/occlusal surfaces of the teeth being radiographed.

- Instruct patients to "slowly close" on the bite block. Align the PID with the aiming ring of the beam alignment device, being careful not to bump the tubehead into the alignment device. This is uncomfortable for patients and may cause some tissue trauma.

Reminders for the Occlusal Technique

- Set the correct exposure factors according to the manufacturer.

- Use a size 4 receptor for this exercise.

CLINICAL LABORATORY ACTIVITY 11-1

Peer Patient Exercises (NO EXPOSURES!)

Objectives

- Demonstrate the correct placement of ½ of a complete series utilizing the bisecting technique; this includes receptor placement, tubehead placement, and correct exposure control settings.

- Demonstrate the correct placement of four bite-wing with tabs projections; this includes receptor placement, tubehead placement, and correct exposure control settings.

- Demonstrate the correct placement of ½ of a complete series utilizing the paralleling technique; this includes receptor placement, tubehead placement, correct exposure control settings, and correct beam alignment device assembly.

- Demonstrate the correct placement of four occlusal projections; this includes receptor placement, tubehead placement, and correct exposure control settings.

Equipment Needed

- radiology cubicle prepared with appropriate infection control protocol

- lead apron and thyroid collar

- receptors in a plastic cup

- beam alignment devices

- disposable bite blocks

- cotton rolls

Procedures

1. Wash hands and don gloves.

2. Place receptors, cup, bite blocks, and cotton rolls on the covered work surface in a radiation-safe area, just outside the radiology cubicle.

3. Turn on the x-ray machine and set the exposure control panel to the appropriate setting for the maxillary canine projection.

4. Take off gloves and wash hands.

5. Greet the "patient," seat in the dental chair, and utilize the lead apron and thyroid collar.

6. Wash hands and re-glove.

7. Follow the appropriate exposure sequences as outlined in previous sections of the manual. Whenever possible, perform procedures under faculty/staff supervision for observation and feedback regarding technique protocol. It is suggested to begin these exercises with the bisecting technique, followed by bite-wings with tabs, paralleling, and occlusal techniques.

12 Paralleling Technique: Peer Patient Complete Mouth Series

CRITERIA FOR COMPETENCY EXAMINATION

Student places a complete series (an average of 18 receptor placements) on a peer patient in 45 minutes or less under faculty/staff observation. No students are exposed to radiation. Receptors are placed intraorally and the position indicating device (PID) is aligned correctly with no exposure.
The complete mouth series includes:

- six or more anterior periapical images

- eight posterior periapical images

- four bite-wing images

Grade is dependent on the following:

- lead apron/thyroid collar placement

- correct exposure sequence

- correct assembly of beam alignment devices

- proper infection control procedures utilized

- correct exposure control settings chosen

- appropriate patient management

- receptor placement

Supervising faculty/staff should also document any obvious errors seen in the procedure, such as noticeable cone-cuts, improper receptor placement, incorrect XCP assembly, patient management issues, and so on. Since no images will be produced, faculty must observe the operators very closely during the complete mouth series.

A competency score of at least 75% is required to pass this examination. If the student does not reach a level of competency, it is at the discretion of the faculty whether the examination may be given a second time.

Image Critique Form
Competency Exam: Peer Patient Complete Mouth Series
Students: Evaluate the images created for this lab session. Use the letters in the Critique Key to describe errors seen on the images. Label each exposure with any errors seen.

Student Name: _____   Patient Name: _____   Date of Exam: _____

Area Exposed	Student Evaluation of Error	Retakes (Y)	Pt Management Issues* (need faculty signature)	Faculty Evaluation of Error*	Critique Key
Max Right Molar					B = exposed backwards
Max Right Premolar					C = cone-cut
Max Right Canine					E = elongation
Max Centrals					F = foreshortening
Max Left Canine					FM = mounting error
Max Left Premolar					H = horizontal angulation
Max Left Molar					IC = infection control error
Right Molar Bite-wing					LA = failure to place lead apron
Right Premolar Bite-wing					M = movement
Left Premolar Bite-wing					Ms = misc (specify)
Left Molar Bite-wing					P = receptor placement
Mand Right Molar					PR = processing (specify)
Mand Right Premolar					R = retake (specify)
Mand Right Canine					FP = Frankfort plane (up/down)
Mand Centrals					FT = focal trough (ant/post)
Mand Left Canine					G = ghost image
Mand Left Premolar					MID = midsagittal plane
Mand Left Molar					LAA = lead apron artifact
PANORAMIC RADIOGRAPH					

Grade Achieved: _____   Faculty Signature: _____

*Faculty: Review the images and critique as necessary; decide if retakes are necessary. Patient management issues may be documented in future semesters.

Image Critique Form
Competency Exam: Peer Patient Complete Mouth Series
Students: Evaluate the images created for this lab session. Use the letters in the Critique Key to describe errors seen on the images. Label each exposure with any errors seen.

Student Name: _____ **Patient Name:** _____ **Date of Exam:** _____

Area Exposed	Student Evaluation of Error	Retakes (Y)	Pt Management Issues* (need faculty signature)	Faculty Evaluation of Error*
Max Right Molar				
Max Right Premolar				
Max Right Canine				
Max Centrals				
Max Left Canine				
Max Left Premolar				
Max Left Molar				
Right Molar Bite-wing				
Right Premolar Bite-wing				
Left Premolar Bite-wing				
Left Molar Bite-wing				
Mand Right Molar				
Mand Right Premolar				
Mand Right Canine				
Mand Centrals				
Mand Left Canine				
Mand Left Premolar				
Mand Left Molar				
PANORAMIC RADIOGRAPH				

Grade Achieved: _____   **Faculty Signature:** _____

Critique Key

B = exposed backwards
C = cone-cut
E = elongation
F = foreshortening
FM = mounting error
H = horizontal angulation
IC = infection control error
LA = failure to place lead apron
M = movement
Ms = misc (specify)
P = receptor placement
PR = processing (specify)
R = retake (specify)
FP = Frankfort plane (up/down)
FT = focal trough (ant/post)
G = ghost image
MID = midsagittal plane
LAA = lead apron artifact

*Faculty: Review the images and critique as necessary; decide if retakes are necessary. Patient management issues may be documented in future semesters.

13 Peer Patient Exercises: Panoramic Technique

BASIC CONCEPTS OF THE PANORAMIC TECHNIQUE

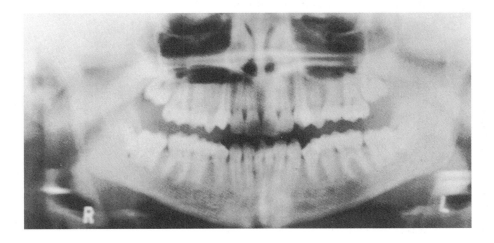

- Infection control protocol must be strictly observed!
- Load the cassette into the panoramic machine according to manufacturer instructions.
- Give instructions on the operation of the machine to the patient.
- Instruct patient to sit or stand erect. It is advisable to adjust the height of the machine according to the patient height before instructing the patient to step in close to the machine.
- Guide the patient into the focal trough; align the midsagittal and Frankfort planes correctly.

CLINICAL LABORATORY ACTIVITY 13-1

Panoramic Peer Patient Exercises (NO EXPOSURES!)

Objectives

- Discuss the purpose and uses of panoramic images.
- Locate the following equipment: panoramic machine on/off switch, machine height adjustment controls, panoramic tubehead, head positioner, location of focal trough, exposure controls, and panoramic cassette.
- Describe the general patient positioning guidelines for exposure of panoramic images.
- Discuss common errors that may occur during exposure of panoramic images.
- Describe advantages and disadvantages of panoramic imaging.

Introduction

The goal of this laboratory exercise is to familiarize the student with the operations of the panoramic machine and surrounding unit. The student will have the opportunity to practice the panoramic technique with a peer patient *without exposure*.

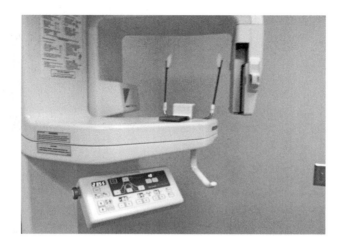

EXAMPLE OF DIAGNOSTIC PANORAMIC IMAGES

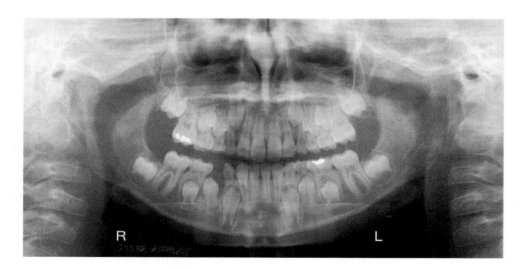

Equipment Needed

- radiology cubicle prepared with appropriate infection control protocol

- lead apron

- bite block with disposable plastic slip

- cassette

- cotton rolls

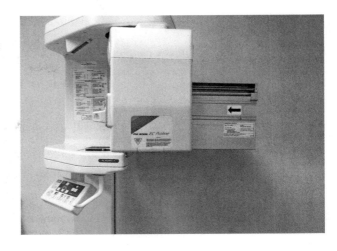

Procedure

1. Turn on the panoramic machine and set the exposure control panel to the appropriate setting for the adult projection.

2. Retrieve cassette with receptor for the panoramic projection from the central dispensing area. Correctly load cassette into the machine. Place cotton rolls on the covered work surface.

3. Cover the bite block with a disposable plastic slip.

4. Greet peer patient and direct him or her into the area near the panoramic machine.

5. Briefly explain the operation of the panoramic machine to the patient and the need to hold extremely still throughout the procedure. Suggest an approximate length of time of exposure (e.g., 20 seconds).

6. Place the lead apron (without the thyroid collar) on the patient and ensure it is low around the patient's neck.

7. Wash hands and don gloves.

8. Instruct patient to remove all metallic objects from the head and neck area. Offer a protected area to contain these objects.

9. Raise or lower the machine to a comfortable height for the patient. Instruct the patient to sit or stand as straight as possible.

10. Place the patient into the focal trough of the machine by guiding their anterior teeth into the grooves on the bite block (Fig. 13-1).

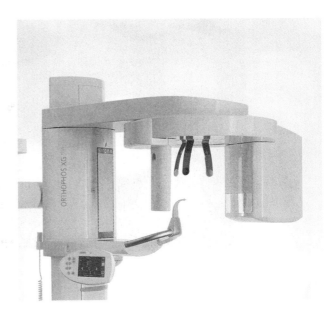

Fig. 13-1. Courtesy of Sirona Dental USA, Charlotte, NC.

11. Position the midsagittal plane perpendicular to the floor.

12. Position the Frankfort plane parallel to the floor.

13. Instruct the patient to swallow and allow his or her tongue to rise to the roof of the mouth.

14. Reinforce that the patient must hold still during the entire exposure.

15. Demonstrate the correct way to exit and dismiss the patient from the panoramic machine.

16. Remove the cassette and complete all infection control procedures, disinfect all surfaces including the bite block, head positioning guides, machine handles, and exposure control switch. Contaminated bite blocks are often placed in a cold sterilizing solution.

17. Extraoral cassettes should be handled with clean, ungloved hands.

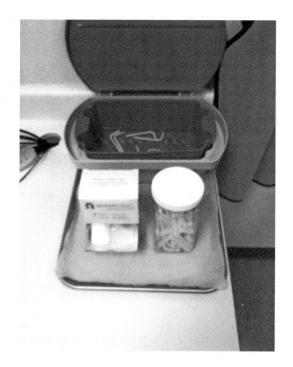

Upon completion of panoramic peer patient exercise and infection control procedures, ask your instructor to check that all procedures have been accomplished correctly.

PROCEDURE STEP	COMPLETED (✓)	STUDENT COMMENTS
1. Turn on the panoramic machine and set the exposure control panel to the appropriate setting for the adult projection.		
2. Retrieve and load into the machine. Place cotton rolls on the covered work surface.		
3. Cover the bite block with a disposable plastic slip		
4-5. Greet patient and explain procedure.		
6. Place apron.		
7. Wash hands and don gloves.		
8. Instruct patient to remove all metallic objects from the head and neck area.		
9. Adjust machine height.		
10. Place patient into the focal trough.		
11. Position the midsagittal plane perpendicular to the floor.		
12. Position the Frankfort plane parallel to the floor.		
13. Instruct the patient to swallow and allow the tongue to rise to the roof of the mouth.		
14. Remind patient to hold still.		
15. Demonstrate the correct manner to exit the machine and dismiss the patient.		
16. Remove the cassette and complete infection control procedures		
17. Handle cassette with clean ungloved hands.		

ASSESSMENT 13-1

Questions for Group Discussion

1. How would you answer a patient who asks a question about radiation dosage from a panoramic exposure?

_____

_____

_____

2. What modifications might be necessary to expose a panoramic image on an edentulous patient?

_____

_____

_____

3. What modification might be necessary to expose a panoramic image on a child that is not tall enough to reach the bite block and head positioning devices?

_____

_____

_____

4. Is a panoramic image a good substitute for a complete intraoral series? Why or why not?

_____

_____

_____

5. What would you say to a patient who cannot remove an intraoral piercing before panoramic exposure?

_____

_____

_____

14 Competency Examination: Peer Patient Panoramic Technique

CRITERIA FOR COMPETENCY EXAMINATION

For this competency examination, students may be placed in groups of three: one student will act as the patient, one will act as the operator, and one will act as the faculty member. Students will then rotate, allowing everyone an opportunity to function in one of these three roles.

Grade will be determined by the "faculty" and is dependent on the following:

- lead apron placement
- clarity of instructions given (includes jewelry removal, proper tongue/lip placements, straight posture, and holding still through entire exposure)
- correct alignment of the patient with the focal trough, Frankfort plane, and midsagittal plane
- proper infection control procedures utilized
- correct exposure control settings chosen
- appropriate patient management and oral instructions for exposure
- proper handling of extraoral cassette and receptor

The "faculty" member should also document any obvious errors seen in the procedure, such as improper loading of receptor, using the thyroid collar, improper patient positioning, and so on.

A competency score of at least 75% is required to pass this examination. If the student does not reach a level of competency, it is at the discretion of the faculty whether the examination may be given a second time.

Image Critique Form
Competency Exam: Peer Patient Panoramic Exercise

Student Name: _____ Patient Name: _____ Date of Exam: _____

Area Exposed	Student Evaluation of Error	Retakes (Y)	Pt Management Issues* (need faculty signature)	Faculty Evaluation of Error*
PANORAMIC RADIOGRAPH				

Critique Key

LA = failure to place lead apron
M = movement
FP = Frankfort plane (up/down)
FT = focal trough (ant/post)
G = ghost image
MID = midsagittal plane
LAA = lead apron artifact
Ms = misc (specify)

Grade Achieved: _____   Faculty Signature: _____

*Faculty: Review the images and critique as necessary; decide if retakes are necessary. Patient management issues may be documented in future semesters.

Image Critique Form
Competency Exam: Peer Patient Panoramic Exercise

Student Name: _____   Patient Name: _____   Date of Exam: _____

Area Exposed	Student Evaluation of Error	Retakes (Y)	Pt Management Issues* (need faculty signature)	Faculty Evaluation of Error*	Critique Key
PANORAMIC RADIOGRAPH					LA = failure to place lead apron M = movement FP = Frankfort plane (up/down) FT = focal trough (ant/post) G = ghost image MID = midsagittal plane LAA = lead apron artifact Ms = misc (specify)

Grade Achieved: _____   Faculty Signature: _____

*Faculty: Review the images and critique as necessary; decide if retakes are necessary. Patient management issues may be documented in future semesters.

482

CONGRATULATIONS!

As the end of the radiology laboratory course draws near, preparation for live patient appointments is quickly approaching. Your faculty will review important documents used in clinic for the treatment of patients who require a radiographic examination. Many documents must be completed and signed by the patient, supervising dentist, and faculty member before exposure of images. Faculty will also review the clinic protocol on radiographic exams, including sign-up sheets and times when radiology cubicles are available.

A few reminders for your first *live* patient in radiology:

BE CONFIDENT! In-depth teaching and training has occurred to prepare you to expose and retrieve diagnostic images. Work efficiently, and take each exposure one at a time.

BE ORGANIZED! Have clinical documents ready, prepare the radiology cubicle accordingly, know the correct exposure sequences, and have all supplies at hand.

BE PREPARED! This may be a new experience for the patient, so be prepared with answers to questions about radiation safety and protection, as well as findings revealed on the images. Ask for assistance from faculty when needed.

Take pride in your work. Exposing diagnostic images for the patient is a critical step in creating the proper treatment plan for future dental care. Congratulations on taking an important step toward your career as a dental health care provider!